CHILD HEALTH IN A
MULTICULTURAL SOCIETY

CHILD HEALTH IN A MULTICULTURAL SOCIETY

JOHN BLACK FRCP

Honorary Consultant Paediatrician
King's College Hospital, London

Published by the British Medical Journal
Tavistock Square, London WC1H 9JR

First edition 1985. Title of 1st edition was "The New
Paediatrics: Child Health in Ethnic Minorities"
Second edition 1989

ISBN 0 7279 0266 0

Filmset and printed in Great Britain by
Latimer Trend & Company Ltd, Plymouth

Contents

FOREWORD TO SECOND EDITION

It is now four years since the articles, which formed the basis of this book, were written. Since then, a number of changes have occurred which have affected the children of the ethnic minority groups in Britain.

The most important change is that, increasingly, the children attending surgeries and clinics have been born to parents who were themselves born in Britain, or were brought up here. The attitudes and expectations of these children are similar to those of their schoolmates, but those who are identifiably "non-white" find themselves obstructed and frustrated by the same barriers of racial prejudice and intolerance as their parents or grandparents. In general, entry into the professions and some occupations has become easier for "non-whites": but barriers remain nevertheless.

On the other hand, there is an increasing appreciation in the National Health Service, at least, of the differing needs of each ethnic group or subgroup, and in most areas better provision for these needs has been made. There is no longer a tendency to write medical articles about "Asians", without regard to geographical origin, genetic make-up, dietary customs, or religion. Information of value on the aetiology of, for example, congenital malformations, diabetes, coronary heart disease, and hypertension, should be obtained from studies comparing the incidence or prevalence of such conditions in the different Asian groups in Britain.

On the debit side, the Health Education Authority is no longer printing some of the multilingual information material which was produced by its predecessor, the Health Education Council. Far from giving a lead in this matter, the Health Education Authority has left it to local branches to produce the appropriate literature, but the necessary local initiative and funding seem to be lacking.

I would like to take this opportunity of thanking the many people who have made constructive suggestions about the content of this book. I have tried to incorporate their ideas in this new edition, and have attempted to bring it up to date.

JOHN BLACK
1989

Acknowledgements

I thank Alix Henley for her help in the preparation of the first three chapters and for permission to use material from her book, "*Asian Patients in Hospital and at Home*", published by Pitman Medical for the King Edward's Hospital Fund for London.

I am also grateful for help and advice to Dr Malcolm Arthurton, formerly consultant paediatrician, Bradford Children's Hospital; Dr Bernadette Modell, University College Hospital, London; Dr J S Gill, department of medicine, University of Birmingham; Dr A G Antoniou, consultant paediatrician, Winchester; Dr S K F Chong, consultant paediatrician, Gravesend; Dr Colin Miller, consultant paediatrician, Warrington; Dr Michael Baraitser, consultant clinical geneticist, The Hospital for Sick Children, London; Dr J C Sharp, clinical pathologist, London; at King's College Hospital, London, Dr Alex Mowat, Dr Margaret Pollak, Dr Mary Horn, and Dr Andrew Lestas; Vanessa Shaw, paediatric dietitian; Andria Suk Min Li, Chinese Community Centre, London; Mr Fuat Memduh, Cyprus Turkish Association, London; Mr George Eugeniou, Cypriot Advice Centre, London; and Mrs Sandra Parfitt for typing the original manuscript and the major alterations to the second edition. I also acknowledge the patience and courtesy shown to me by parents and children of many different communities in Britain: they have taught me a great deal and have helped me to a better understanding of their problems.

1 The difficulties of living in Britain

An ethnic minority is a group of individuals who consider themselves separate from the general population, and are seen by the population at large to be distinct because of one or more of the following: common geographical or racial origin, skin colour, language, religious beliefs and practices, or dietary customs. Generally such minority groups live in fairly well defined areas in our cities and large towns. The term Asian is used to describe people from the Indian subcontinent and also those who, though originally from India, entered Britain from east Africa. The South East Asian minorities considered here are the Chinese and Vietnamese. In working with families of the various ethnic minorities in Britain doctors and others should avoid "stereotyping" and appreciate that each individual's responses and adaptations to Britain are unique.

Why the children are important

Britain has a long history of acceptance, with varying degrees of tolerance, of peaceful immigration from different parts of Europe, and Italian, Greek, and Cypriot communities have been established in Britain for many generations. Immigration from outside Europe on a large scale is something new and has brought with it problems that were previously unfamiliar to the health services. Even now there is still inadequate instruction about the needs and diseases of minority groups in our medical and nursing schools. The medical and nursing professions have little knowledge of their cultures, religion, and dietary customs, though these often have a direct bearing on medical conditions in the children, and there is a poor appreciation of the difficulties that many families face in adapting to life in Britain.

1

It is often through its children that a family first comes into contact with the medical services, and the family's subsequent attitude to medical care may be determined by the amount of tolerance and understanding which it receives over its children from doctors, nurses, and non-medical staff. Members of the groups that are the subject of these chapters have a high incidence of conditions which do not occur, or are rare, in the general population of the United Kingdom. Most of these conditions, particularly those of genetic or nutritional origin, become apparent in infancy and childhood. Tuberculosis and the tropical and subtropical infections and parasitic infestations are often acquired in childhood. Finally, emotional and behaviour disorders in the children are often a symptom of difficulties in adjustment which the whole family is experiencing.

Types of disease

Genetically determined disease

In some groups genetically determined disease occurs with sufficient frequency and severity to constitute an important health problem—for example, sickle cell anaemia in the Afro-Caribbean community occurs in about 1 in every 400 children born. β Thalassaemia in the Greek, Cypriot, and Italian communities is now much less common than it was a few years ago, due to screening in antenatal clinics and fetal diagnosis of the homozygous state. Similarly, glucose-6-phosphate dehydrogenase deficiency occurs in the Afro-Caribbean, African, Mediterranean, Chinese, and Vietnamese communities but rarely causes serious problems in the United Kingdom except when neonatal jaundice occurs.

In communities where marriages between first or second cousins are common, as in Moslems from Asia, other recessively determined disorders occur with a much greater frequency than in a population where such marriages are rare. Most of these conditions are metabolic disorders, which usually become apparent in the neonatal period or early infancy, though there also appears to be an increased incidence of multiple congenital malformations, which are probably of genetic origin. Homozygous β thalassaemia (major) is relatively common in Moslems from Pakistan.

Acquired diseases

Among people of Asian origin nutritional disorders such as iron deficiency anaemia and rickets manifest themselves in infancy or childhood, and tuberculosis is relatively common in both adults and children. Diseases of the tropics and subtropics, such as malaria and worm and intestinal infestations, are all seen in Asian children who have lived in or visited the Indian subcontinent. Established rheumatic heart disease may be found in the older children of any of the immigrant groups.

Alternative or "indigenous" medicines and traditional practices

Obscure or puzzling symptoms may be due to the effect of medicines sold over the counter or prescribed by unqualified practitioners in the community. Physical methods of treatment, such as "coin rubbing" or cauterisation produce lesions that may be attributed to child abuse, while in Asian children the application round the eyes of cosmetics (surma) that contain lead may expose the child to the risk of lead poisoning.

Diseases related to poor socioeconomic conditions

Low wages, long working hours, and night shift working are common in families from Asia and the Caribbean, and overcrowding and bad housing result in a high incidence of respiratory and gastrointestinal infections. If both parents are working the children may become emotionally and socially deprived if left with a baby minder.

Problems of adaptation and their effect on the children

Cultural shock may develop after a family arrives in Britain, with a severity which is related to the amount of change experienced, and may be initiated by unsympathetic or degrading immigration procedures and exacerbated by difficulties in obtaining accommodation or employment. Adult members of the family may develop a confusional state, paranoid attitudes or behaviour, or depression, causing the children to become anxious and in-

3

secure because of the altered behaviour of their parents. Cultural shock may be succeeded by more permanent states of mind, such as suspiciousness, feelings of insecurity, fear of persecution, or physical violence. Fortunately, in most groups there is usually considerable support available from the rest of their own community or from family members already established in the United Kingdom. At the moment few children are arriving as immigrants, apart from those, mainly from Pakistan and Bangladesh, who are joining their fathers already established in Britain. The Vietnamese "Boat People," without any established community to help them, suffered severely when they settled in Britain.

Insecurity—Insecurity in the parents may manifest itself by a constant anxiety about the health of their children, requiring repeated reassurance, numerous referrals, and requests for investigations and second opinions. There is often a tendency to magnify the child's symptoms. Anxiety about poor weight gain or small stature may indicate a desire that the child, especially a boy, should become as tall and strong as possible to cope with a socially and physically hostile environment. Other signs of parental insecurity include an undue concern about recurrent upper respiratory infections in their children, though this is sometimes simply due to a failure to appreciate that such infections are as inevitable in Britain as are gastrointestinal infections in Asia or Africa.

Reasons for coming to Britain—It is helpful to have some idea of the reason (which is usually the same in each group) why the family came to Britain, since this may influence their readiness to adapt to life in this country. Groups who maintain strong links with their home by frequent visits and live in a closely knit community with its own shops and organisations may not need to alter their way of life very much. Those who have been forced to leave their country because of political, racial, or religious persecution are more likely to have to accept the reality of permanent residence here because they may have little prospect of returning. In most cases families have come to Britain from areas with a depressed or declining economy and few opportunities to improve their standards of living. At the time when most recent immigration occurred, between 1950 and 1970, Britain offered such opportunities, but with the present high level of unemployment many families from Asia and the Caribbean have the worst housing and poor prospects of employment for their children.

4

Divided families—Marital difficulties and emotional upsets in the children may arise when families are split up, often for years, while the father establishes himself in a job or in business in Britain, or there is a delay in obtaining an entry permit. Children born to a couple in their 40s who have been separated for some years may suffer from the rigidity of outlook which often occurs in older than average parents.

Concept of illness and disease—The idea of follow up appointments and long term treatment does not come easily to families from countries where disease is treated episode by episode or only when a crisis occurs. Attendance at follow up appointments may be difficult for many Asian families, partly for these reasons and partly because the mother may be unwilling or unable to bring the child on her own, while the father may not want to risk losing his job by repeatedly taking time off work. Particularly when discussing genetically determined disease or mental retardation, and in giving advice, the help of someone with the same cultural and religious background as the family may be required.

The child's problems

Pressure to succeed—Parental pressure to succeed is often considerable, particularly in those groups which came to Britain with high financial expectations or where, as in the Asians from east Africa, the father has been unable to obtain a job of the status equivalent to that which he left. The child may respond by school refusal or by difficult behaviour at home or at school, particularly when he or she is unable to live up to the parents' hopes or expectations.

Poor school progress may be due to linguistic difficulties at school entry and may be an acute problem in an older child who has recently come to Britain. In families who run restaurants the children may be expected to help behind the scenes instead of doing their homework.

Transcultural problems—Older children, particularly teenagers, often have difficulty in reconciling the patterns of behaviour which they learn at school with those required of them at home. Asian girls may be expected to stay at home in the evenings and not go out to discos. The prospect of an arranged marriage can be deeply disturbing to a girl brought up in the United Kingdom. Children who can be instantly categorised as being "non-European" because of skin colour or facial appearance may have great difficulty in establishing their true identity and gaining acceptance in the community as a whole.

Further reading

Arthurton M W. Immigrant children and the day-to-day work of a paediatrician. *Arch Dis Child* 1972; **47**:126–30.

Arthurton M W. Some medical problems of Asian immigrant children. *Maternal and Child Health* 1977; **2**:316–21.

Fuller J H, Toon P D. *Medical practice in a multicultural society*. Oxford: Heinemann Professional Publishing, 1988.

Kirkwood K, Herbertson M A, Packes A S. Biosocial aspects of ethnic minorities. *Journal of Biosocial Science*. 1983; suppl 8: 1–225.

King's Fund Centre. Ethnic minorities and health care in London. London: King's Fund Centre, 1982. (A list of local projects and initiatives concerning ethnic minorities available from the centre, 126 Albert Street, London NW1.)

Lobo E de H. *Children of immigrants in Britain, their health and social problems*. London: Hodder and Stoughton, 1978.

Pollak M. The care of immigrant children. In: Hart C, ed. *Child care in general practice*. 2nd ed. Edinburgh: Churchill Livingstone, 1982.

Runnymede Trust and the Radical Statistics Group. *Britain's black population*. Guildford, Surrey: Heinemann Educational Books, 1978.

Sampson C. *The neglected ethic; religious and cultural factors in the care of patients*. London: McGraw-Hill, 1982.

Tajfel H. *Social psychology of minorities*. London: Minority Rights Group. Undated. (Report No 38.)

Useful addresses

Joint Council for the Welfare of Immigrants,
115 Old Street
London EC1V 9JR

01 251 8706

2 Contact with the health services

Naming systems and religions

To have one's name mispronounced or misspelt is annoying and a loss of personal dignity. Receptionists in general practice, hospital record clerks, and also doctors and nurses should receive instruction in the correct pronunciation of the commoner names of the ethnic groups in their area. They also need to understand the naming systems since embarrassment and confusion can be caused by incorrect use, and a satisfactory system for recording names reduces the number of lost or duplicated records. In general the names of people of Afro-Caribbean or Mediterranean origin do not cause problems, their naming systems being similar to British ones, but the naming systems of Asians, Moslems, and Chinese are very different, although some families change the patterns of their names to conform to British practice. Leaflets are available giving the correct pronunciation of the commoner Asian names and explaining the various systems of naming which are in use (pages 16 and 17).

Religion should be recorded in every case, as the religious beliefs of the parents and children must be respected, and dietary restrictions observed when the child is in hospital.

Information

Instruction leaflets—In areas where one or more linguistic groups form a significant proportion of the population notices should be written in the appropriate script and language. Dietary instruction and information leaflets about the use of enuresis alarms, inhalers,

7

etc, should also be made available in these languages. It cannot be assumed that all Asians are literate in their own language, however, but people who can read their own language can usually also read English.[1] For the illiterate there is no substitute for the spoken word. The useful but poorly publicised booklets, such as *Your Right to Health in Great Britain* in 12 languages, which was published by the Health Education Council, are no longer produced by its successor, the Health Education Authority.

Interpreters—In some practices and hospitals, staff may be readily available to act as interpreters, but when this is not so, or if the parents speak an unusual language or dialect, special arrangements for an interpreter should be made. In some cities interpreter services have been set up. Except in emergencies, there is no excuse for failing to obtain an adequate history because of linguistic difficulties, and the parents should have the opportunity of explaining what they feel is wrong with their child; they also deserve a full explanation of the child's illness. Without a proper understanding of what is wrong and what is required, cooperation with treatment will be unsatisfactory. In general it is not helpful to use older children as interpreters, particularly when the parents find it embarrassing to discuss their problems in front of their own child.

Local contacts—It is useful to have a list of local community leaders, religious or otherwise, who can be consulted over difficult problems, particularly when ethical considerations are involved. In areas with a large community having a common religion it is useful to have a local "priest" appointed as a chaplain to the hospital group—for example, an Imam for the local Moslem community.

Surgery and clinic times—Since non-attendance at clinics is often due to the reluctance of an English speaking father or elder sibling to take time off work for fear of losing his job, the setting up of evening clinics should be considered; this, of course, applies to any parents who have difficulty in attending during the morning or afternoon. Such evening clinics or surgeries might reduce attendance at the accident and emergency department of the local hospital.

Seeing the doctor

The history

It is essential to gain the confidence of the parents and child, and this can be done only by taking an unhurried approach. It is easy, especially if there is difficulty in understanding what the parents are saying, or vice versa, for the doctor to become baffled and impatient and to give the impression that he thinks the parents are ignorant, stupid, or overanxious. Patience and a sympathetic attitude, without condescension, will gain the confidence of confused and anxious parents.

In addition to the usual history the following information may be helpful in understanding the family's background:

(*a*) country of origin of the parents: how long have they been in Britain?

(*b*) languages spoken: first language, others;

(*c*) place of birth of the child: if born outside the UK, how long has the child been in this country?

(*d*) has the child visited the parents' home country? If so, for how long and when was the last visit? Did the child become ill while on any of the visits and if so what treatment was given, and did the child receive any injections (risk of hepatitis B)?

(*e*) are the parents related?

(*f*) the extended family: how many adults or children other than the parents and their children are there in the household?

Heights and weights—Centile charts for the heights and weights of the children of some ethnic groups have been constructed for children living in parts of Asia and Africa, but they are of limited value for children born and brought up in Britain. Since it is the pattern of growth or weight gain which is usually more important than the height or weight on any one occasion, deviation from the centile lines can be appreciated quite satisfactorily by using the standard Tanner and Whitehouse charts for British children.

The examination—A child often senses the anxiety and insecurity of the parents on a visit to the doctor or hospital, and a clumsy or hurried attempt to get him or her completely undressed may upset both the parents and the child. Asian girls, particularly Moslems, may object to being fully undressed or to being examined by a man. In the absence of acute illness it is often better to

9

arrange for a return visit on a day when a woman can carry out the physical examination. When a girl has to be examined by a man, permission for this should be obtained from the accompanying adult.

Particular care should be taken in prescribing drugs or investigations via the rectal route, as the use of the rectum is deeply offensive to Asians. Similarly, if a rectal examination is necessary the reason for doing it should be fully explained.

Diagnostic difficulties and skin pigmentation

In infants of Asian, south east Asian, or African origin the inappropriately named "Mongolian blue spot" may be mistaken for a bruise, and child abuse may be wrongly suspected. The "blue spot" is usually confined to the sacral area but may extend into the posterior thoracic and scapular regions or along the posterior part of the thighs. It is also seen in children whose parents come from the Mediterranean area and is occasionally seen in infants of very dark haired indigenous white parents. In all racial groups the blue-black pigmentation gradually disappears by the age of 18 months to 2 years.

Skin pigmentation may prevent anaemia, cyanosis, or jaundice from being immediately obvious, and rashes may be difficult to detect. Anaemia should cause no real difficulty if the conjunctiva, the oral mucosa, and the palms and soles are examined. Peripheral cyanosis is easily missed, but other observations, such as capillary refilling after pressure, temperature of the tip of the nose and big toe, heart rate, and blood pressure, should all be recorded if shock is suspected. Central cyanosis is easily detected by examining the tongue and oral mucosa.

Jaundice, particularly in the newborn, is easily missed in the mature infant with a dark skin,[3] but immature infants of Asian or African origin often have light skins in the first few weeks of life. In the dark skinned infant the doctor should attempt to examine the sclerae, but this is difficult in the newborn, and the colour of the palms and soles can be assessed after blanching by light pressure. The hard palate and fraenum of the tongue should also be examined and the gums can be blanched by pressure with a spoon or spatula.

Rashes, particularly those due to rubella and measles, may cause difficulty, but the presence of enlarged occipital glands is helpful in confirming rubella. In malnourished children who have recently come to Britain measles may be unexpectedly severe, with a confluent or occasionally haemorrhagic rash; however, in the first two days after the appearance of the rash Koplik's spots may still be visible in the mouth.

Particularly in Asians, emotional or psychological disorders may be presented to the doctor in the form of apparent organic symptoms, such as headache, backache, limb pains, or "fever." It is usually advisable to do one or two organically orientated investigations initially; otherwise the parents may not feel that their child's symptoms have been taken seriously.

The child in hospital

Children, particularly of preschool age, are often very unhappy in hospital, where there may be no member of the ward staff who knows their language. The child who speaks no English may be socially ignored by medical and nursing staff, who find the effort to communicate too frustrating or time consuming. The mother may have difficulty in visiting in the morning or afternoon if she is not accustomed to using public transport unaccompanied by her husband or a male relative. Hospital staff must be sensitive to the various problems which may arise in relation to diet, clothes, the wearing of jewellery or objects of religious significance, and the taking of blood. An explanation of the purpose of an operation may require the help of an interpreter. Rules about bringing food into hospital should be relaxed if the hospital cannot supply a diet in accordance with the parents' religious beliefs; it is very important to ill and lonely children in unfamiliar surrounding to be given food which looks and tastes familiar. In many countries it is the custom for the mother to sleep in the same room, or in the same bed, as her sick child. When the mother obviously wishes to sleep in the same bed as her child the hospital should provide an appropriately sized bed; there is no excuse for the sight of a mother who has squeezed herself into a child's cot.

1 Aslam M, Davis S S, Fletcher R. Compliance in medication by Asian immigrants. *Nursing Times* 1979; 75:931–2.

2 Cook S. The agony of putting pain into words. *Guardian* 1983; May 18:11.
3 Tarnow-Mordi W O, Pickering D. Missed jaundice in black infants; a hazard. *Br Med J* 1983; **286**:463–4.

Further reading

Mares P, Henley A, Baxter C. *Health care in multiracial Britain*. Cambridge: National Extension College, 1985.

3 Asian families I: cultures

This chapter considers the problems of children whose families have originated directly from India, Pakistan, and Bangladesh and indirectly from the Indian subcontinent via east Africa.

The extended family is of great importance in Asian culture. It consists of three generations: the husband (head of the family) and wife, their sons and wives, and their children. In Britain the traditional roles of husband and family cannot always be sustained; the husband may feel that his authority has diminished and may worry because his children do not look to the extended family in Asia. His wife may feel isolated at home, lacking the support of relatives, and may see her husband and children, with their contacts outside the home, adapting better to life in Britain. The children will attempt, with varying degrees of success, to cope with life in two cultures. Most Asian parents in Britain approve of arranged marriages and their children usually accept them as marriage is very much a family affair.

The three main religions

Hinduism

Except for the Sikhs from the Punjab, a few Moslems and Christians, Indian families are Hindus, as are most Indian families from east Africa. In Britain distinctions of caste have less importance than in India, though marriages usually occur within the same caste. Marriage is regarded as a sacrament; divorce, though rare, is becoming more common among Hindus in Britain. There is no religious prohibition against postmortem examinations, but the reasons for carrying out this investigation should be fully and tactfully explained to the family, as such a request may be completely unexpected. After death the family may want to wash the body and are often particular about who touches it. The body is cremated, but children may be buried.

Hindus do not eat beef and are usually vegetarian, though the strictness of observance varies greatly. Gujarati Hindus are usually very strict vegetarians.

Parents may put jewellery of religious importance on their children before they go into hospital; these articles of jewellery should not be removed without the parents' consent.

Sikhism

All Sikhs come originally from the Punjab, though many have come to Britain from east Africa. Those who observe their religion strictly wear the five signs:

(*a*) uncut hair of the head and body (kes, pronounced kesh) for both men and women;

(*b*) a comb (khanga) to secure the hair on the head; men wear a turban over this. The wearing of turbans has caused difficulties with legislation when crash helmets must be worn and also in some schools. Boys do not wear turbans until the age of 10–12 years, and before this they secure their hair in a knot on top of the head with a small cloth (rumal);

(*c*) a metal bracelet (kara) worn on the right wrist by both men and women; this must *never* be removed, even after death;

(*d*) a special undergarment (kacch, pronounced kaccha) for men only; in Britain ordinary underpants are often worn instead;

(*e*) a small symbolic dagger (kirpan or khanda) worn by both sexes, often as a brooch or pendant. It is occasionally and mistakenly regarded as an offensive weapon by some headteachers, who have attempted to prohibit its wearing in school; in hospital also, failure to understand the importance of the kirpan has result in its forcible removal, to the great distress of the patient and family.

As in Hinduism marriage is regarded as a sacrament, and divorce, though possible, is not approved but is becoming more common in Britain.

14

There is no prohibition against necropsies. After death the body is cremated.

Most Sikhs will eat pork but not beef; in general, however, they rarely eat meat. Their diet is nevertheless usually well balanced, and the children are well nourished.

Islam

The Mosque is the centre of male religious and community life for Moslems and is in the charge of an Imam. Physical seclusion (purdah) for women was prescribed by Mohammed, but the degree of observance of purdah and the wearing of a cover over the face vary considerably. Marriage is a civil contract, not a sacrament; in Britain it is rare for a Moslem man from the Indian subcontinent to have more than one wife; divorce is permitted but not approved. Moslem boys must be circumcised before puberty; as with Jewish circumcision this cannot normally be done under the National Health Service unless there is a medical indication for the operation; however some paediatric surgeons prefer to do circumcisions under the National Health Service rather than have to deal with the complications of an unskilled operation, since in many areas there is a shortage of skilled Moslem practitioners.

According to Islamic law the body must be buried within 24 hours of death, but full observance of all the rules may be difficult in Britain. After death no part of the body may be removed or damaged in any way. Necropsies should therefore be performed only when there is a legal requirement, as ordered by the coroner; the need for these must be fully explained to the parents. After death the body is buried and must not be cremated.

Dietary observances are strictly prescribed by Islamic law. Meat must be "halal"—that is, the animal must have been killed in a specific way. No Moslem will eat pork, pork products, or anything that contains pork or pig derivatives; if there is any doubt about the origin or content of a food they will refuse it.

Names

Each of the three religions has a differnt naming system. The same name may be spelt in a number of different ways, often

TABLE I—*Hindu naming system*

	First name (personal, usually different male and female names)	Middle or complementary name (different male and female names)	Subcaste name
Female	Arima	Devi	Patel
Male	Naresh	Lal	Chopra

within the same family or by the same person on different occasions. Record clerks and receptionists should be taught to record Asian names in a standardised manner.

Hindu naming system—Hindus have a first or personal name, a middle or complementary name, and a subcaste or family name, which in Britain is used as a surname. The husband's subcaste name is adopted by the wife on marriage and is used by the children (table I). Both first and middle or complementary names should be used together; sometimes they are written as one word—for example, Arimadevi. In Gujarati families the middle name is usually the father's first name, to distinguish between different families all called Patel/Shah, or other common subcaste names.

Sikh naming system—The Sikh system is based on the Hindu system. In rural India the subcaste names have been abandoned, but in Britain they may be readopted and used as a surname. If the subcaste name is not used Singh may be used as a surname. All Sikh men have the complementary (or middle) name of Singh (meaning lion) and all Sikh women the complementary name of Kaur (meaning princess) (table II). The Sikh first name is used by family and friends, whereas for polite use, as in the outpatient department or surgery, the first and complementary names are used, followed by the subcaste name if used. The subcaste name is adopted by the wife on marriage and is used by the children. Some families simply use Singh as the surname for all male members and Kaur as the surname for all female members of the family. As this

TABLE II—*Sikh naming system*

	First name (personal name, male and female names usually the same)	Middle or complementary (religious) name	(Subcaste name)
Female	Jaswinder	(all women) Kaur	(Gill)
Male	Armarjit	(all men) Singh	(Bamra)

is confusing a reasonable attempt should be made to discover the subcaste name, to simplify the filing of records.

Moslem naming system—Moslems from different parts of the world have different naming systems. In those from the Indian subcontinent or of Asian origin from east Africa there are traditionally no names shared by the whole family; and wives and children do not adopt the husband's name. Moslem men have two or more names, one being a personal name and the other given first, often has a religious connection, such as Mohammed (sometimes abbreviated to Moh'd) or Ali. In polite or formal use the man is addressed by his full name—for example, Mohammed Habibur Rahman. In Britain families usually use a clan name such as Chaudry or Khan as the surname. Women have a personal name followed either by a title that is more or less equivalent to Ms (Begum, Bibi) or by a second name: formally the woman is addressed by her names followed by the title. The record clerk should always ask for the husband's or father's family name (table III).

Different Asian groups in Britain

With the exception of those from east Africa the reason for emigration of most Asians has been economic—that is, a desire to improve the economic conditions of the family—especially when the economic conditions in the home country are poor, bad, or deteriorating. Asians in east Africa were expelled, or life was made so uncomfortable that they left. Table IV shows the main groups of Asians in Britain from India, east Africa, and Pakistan.

TABLE III—*Moslem naming system and way of recording it*

Name	Record as:
Husband	
Mohammed Habibur Rahman	(Mohammed) Habibur RAHMAN
Wife	
Jameela Katoon	Jameela Katoon, wife of Mohammed Habibur RAHMAN
Son	
Shafiur Mia	Shafiur Mia, son of Mohammed Habibur RAHMAN
Daughter	
Shameema Bibi	Shameema Bibi, daughter of Mohammed Habibur RAHMAN

TABLE IV—*Main groups from India, east Africa, and Pakistan*

People from:	are called:	their religion is:	their first language is:	they may speak some:	they first settled in:
India and east Africa					
Gujarat: south and central regions	Gujaratis	Hinduism, a few Islam	Gujarati	Hindi	*Gujarati Hindus:* Birmingham, Leicester, N London, Preston, SE England, Wellingborough, W Bromwich, W Midlands
Gujarat: north region, Kutch	Kutchis or Gujaratis	Hinduism, a few Islam	Kuchi or Gujarati	Gujarati, Hindi	*Gujarati Moslems:* Bolton, Leicester, Preston, Tameside, Wandsworth
The Punjab state	Punjabis (Sikh)	Sikhism	Punjabi	Hindi	Birmingham, Chatham, Gravesend, Rochester, Leeds, Maidenhead, Southampton, Warwick, Leamington Spa, W London, W Midlands
	Punjabis (non-Sikh)	Hinduism	Punjabi	Hindi	
Other parts of India* (Bombay, Delhi, etc)	Indians, or name of state	Hinduism	Hindi	English	London and other large cities
East Africa, Kenya, Malawi, Tanzania, Uganda, Zambia	East African Asians	Hinduism, Islam, or Sikhism, depending on family origins	Gujarati or Punjabi, according to origin	Hindi, English, Swahili	Birmingham, Croydon, Leicester, Loughborough, N and S London, SE England
Pakistan					
The Punjab province	Punjabis	Islam	Punjabi	Urdu	Bedford, Glasgow, High Wycombe, Humberside, Lancashire
Mirpur district (in Azad Kashmir)	Mirpuris	Islam	Mirpuri (Punjabi dialect)	Punjabi, Urdu	Maidenhead, Sheffield, Slough, W Midlands, W Yorkshire
North West Frontier	Pathans (phonetically Pataans)	Islam	Pashto	Punjabi, Urdu	

*A few families who came originally from Goa are Roman Catholics and usually have names of Portuguese origin, such as de Silva

18

TABLE V—*Women's dress*

	Hindus	Moslems from Pakistan or Gujarat, Sikhs from the Punjab	Moslems from Bangladesh (Bengalis)
Women	Blouse, sari, and long petticoat	Kameez (tunic), shalwar (trousers), and dupatta or chuni (scarf)	Blouse, sari, and long petticoat (end of sari serves as veil)
Girls	Knee length dress or trousers	Kameez (tunic), shalwar (trousers), and dupatta or chuni (scarf)	Knee length dress or trousers

Gujarat—Apart from a few Moslems the Gujaratis are Hindus. In Britain the men and boys usually wear Western style street clothes. Older women and some girls tend to dress traditionally in blouse, sari, and long petticoat (table V). Hindus from other parts of India dress similarly.

Punjab (Sikhs)—The Sikhs come from the state of Punjab in India (not to be confused with the Moslem province of Punjab in Pakistan); a few come from east Africa. The adult men are distinguished by their turban and beard; boys wear their hair in a knot on top of their heads. Traditional dress of women is a tunic, trousers, and scarf (table V).

Pakistan—Most families from Pakistan come from the province of Punjab, Mirpur (Azad Kashmir), and the North West Frontier province (table IV). They are all Moslems. The men may wear a high collared coat and some type of brimless, often fur, hat; women dress similarly to Sikhs (table V). They emigrated from Pakistan for economic reasons. Difficulties have arisen in physical education classes and games at some schools because the girls are not allowed to expose their legs and arms and cannot wear gym tunics or swimming costumes. Most schools have reached a compromise by allowing the girls to retain their trousers for games and by arranging single sex swimming lessons. Their diet is usually satisfactory, and dietary deficiencies are not common in their children (table VI).

Bangladesh—Most families come from the district of Sylhet; though sometimes known as Bangladeshis, they usually call themselves Bengalis and speak Bengali (usually the Sylheti dialect) as their first language but may speak a little Urdu. They are Moslems. The men dress similarly to the Moslems from Pakistan, but

19

TABLE VI—*Regional diets of main Asian groups in Britain*

	From the Indian Punjab		From Gujarat	From Gujarat	From Pakistan	From Bangladesh
	Sikhs	Hindus	Hindus	Moslems	Moslems	Moslems
Staple source of cereal	Chapatis	Chapatis	Chapatis, rice	Chapatis, rice	Chapatis	Rice
Cooking oil	Ghee*	Ghee	Groundnut oil, some ghee	Groundnut oil, some ghee	Ghee or groundnut oil	Groundnut oil, some ghee
Meat	No beef, rarely pork Some are vegetarians. Most eat chicken or mutton	No beef, usually no pork Mostly vegetarians	No beef, usually no pork Mostly vegetarians	No pork products, halal meat only (usually chicken or mutton)	No pork products, halal meat only (usually chicken or mutton)	No pork products, halal meat only (usually chicken or mutton)
Fish	Occasionally	No	No	Occasionally	Occasionally	Fresh or dried fish often
Eggs	Not a major part of diet	Not eaten by strict vegetarians	Not eaten by strict vegetarians	Usually hard boiled or fried	Usually hard boiled or fried	Usually hard boiled or fried
Dairy products	Very important. Yoghurt, buttermilk, homemade cream cheese, milk (boiled and sweetened)	Very important. Yoghurt, buttermilk, homemade cream cheese, milk (boiled and sweetened)	Important, especially yoghurt and milk (boiled and sweetened)	Fairly important	Fairly important. Yoghurt and milk (boiled and sweetened)	Little or none
Pulses and dahl†	Major source of protein	May be only source of protein	May be almost only source of protein	Fairly important	A few pulses, some dahl	A few pulses, some dahl
Vegetables	Vegetable curries, occasional salad, fresh fruit	Vegetable curries, occasional salad, fresh fruit	Vegetable curries, occasional salad, fresh fruit	Vegetable curries, occasional salad, fresh fruit	Vegetable curries, occasional salad, fresh fruit	Vegetable curries, occasional salad, fresh fruit

*Ghee is clarified butter. †Dahl is the split seed of leguminous vegetables, various sorts of pea, or gram

20

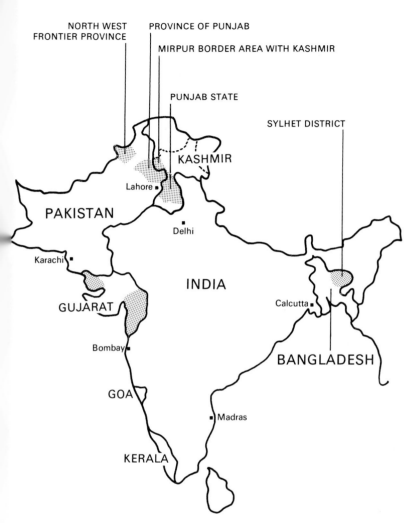

NORTH WEST
FRONTIER PROVINCE

PROVINCE OF PUNJAB

MIRPUR BORDER AREA WITH KASHMIR

PUNJAB STATE

SYLHET DISTRICT

KASHMIR

Lahore ■

PAKISTAN

Delhi ■

Karachi ■

INDIA

GUJARAT

Calcutta ■

Bombay ■

BANGLADESH

GOA

■ Madras

KERALA

Main areas in India, Pakistan and Bangladesh from which immigrants have come (reproduced with permission of author and publishers from Henley, A. Asian patients in hospital and at home, *London, King Edward's Hospital Fund for London, Pitman Medical 1979).*

women dress more like Hindu women, with saris (table V). These families originally settled in Bolton, Bradford, Dundee, east and north east London, Keighley, Luton, Oldham, Scunthorpe, Sheffield, and Tameside; the largest settlement is in Tower Hamlets

21

(east London). The children's diet is often inadequate in iron (due to the late introduction of solids or cereals), vitamin D, and total calories. Children who arrived recently from Bangladesh are often severly undernourished and should be carefully screened for anaemia, worms, and tuberculosis. Their staple cereal is rice, and they eat chicken or mutton (halal), and fresh and dried fish but few dairy products (table VI).

Further reading

Henley A. *Asian patients in hospital and at home.* London: Pitman Medical, 1979.
Wright C. Pakistani family life in Newcastle. *Maternal and Child Health* 1981; **6:**427–30.
Henley A. Asians in Britain: caring for Hindus and their families: religious aspects of care (1983).
Henley A. Asians in Britain: caring for Sikhs and their families: religious aspects of care (1983).
Henley A. Asians in Britain: caring for Muslims and their families: religious aspects of care (1982).
All the above are obtainable from the National Extension College, 18 Brooklands Avenue, Cambridge CB2 2HN (0223-63465/316644).

Further information

The following booklet, published for the DHSS and the King Edward's Hospital Fund for London by the the National Extension College, is available from the college, 16 Brooklands Avenue, Cambridge CB2 2HH: *Asians in Britain: Recording and Using Asian names.*
Other related literature is also available, including guides to the pronunciation of the commoner Hindu, Sikh, and Moslem names with flow charts for records clerks.

4 Asian families II: conditions that may be found in the children

Genetically determined conditions

Blood diseases

β *Thalassaemia* is widely distributed throughout the Indian sub-continent, particularly in the north, though it is not nearly so common as in the Mediterranean area. More cases of homozygous β thalassaemia (thalassaemia major) are now seen in Pakistani families in London than in Greek, Cypriot, and Italian communities (for further discussion on β thalassaemia see chapter 5: Families from the Mediterranean and Aegean). Moslem parents have more difficulty in accepting the ideas of genetic advice, antenatal testing, and termination of pregnancy than have parents from the Mediterranean areas, but the situation is improving.

Haemoglobin D disease may occur in combination with β thalassaemia in children from northern India or Pakistan, and haemoglobin E thalassaemia occurs in Bengalis from Bangladesh. Both of these combined blood disorders result in chronic haemolytic anaemia with splenomegaly, requiring the same sort of treatment as homozygous β thalassaemia.

Sickle cell disease is not common in those groups that have emigrated to Britain; when sickle cell anaemia does occur, it appears to be less severe than in Afro-Caribbeans or Africans. There are also small areas with notable incidence of sickle cell trait in the Nilgiri Hills in South India, Maharashtra, Bihar, Uttar Pradesh and West Bengal[1] (for further discussion on sickle cell disease see chapter 7: Afro-Caribbean and African families).

Glucose-6-phosphate dehydrogenase deficiency is fairly common throughout the northern part of the Indian subcontinent. (B

23

Modell, personal communication, gives an overall incidence of 7% hemizygous males in the Indian subcontinent). The possibility of such a deficiency should always be considered in cases of neonatal jaundice when blood groups are compatible and in any cases of severe and sudden haemolytic anaemia that develop during an acute illness or as a result of taking certain drugs (for further discussion see later chapters). When practicable G6PD deficiency should be excluded before giving primaquine for malaria. Two recent papers,[2][3] based on neonatal screening have shown a higher incidence of congenital hypothyroidism in Asian than in white families. The frequency of consanguineous marriages was high (55% in one study) but the increased number of cases in the Asian group was mainly due to dysgenesis (aplastic, hypoplastic, or ectopic glands), rather than inborn errors of hormone synthesis as might have been expected.

Recessively determined metabolic disorders

There is little doubt that the high incidence of recessively determined metabolic disorders and some of the more unusual malformations in Moslem families from Pakistan is due to the number of marriages among first and second cousins.

Consanguinity

Consanguineous marriage is common in the Pakistani[4] and Bangladeshi communities, but not among the Hindus and Sikhs. The influence of consanguinity on the pattern of disease is still uncertain, and the custom of marriage between first and second cousins should not be condemned by non-Asians. However, a consanguineous marriage does increase the chance of rare inborn errors of metabolism, and possibly of unusual recessively determined malformations, in the offspring. In practical terms, the risk to parents who are first cousins of producing a child with a genetically determined condition, though increased, is still genetically acceptable. The real difficulty arises when a severely malformed or handicapped child is born in a consanguineous marriage and cannot be fitted into any known syndrome, and the chromosomes are normal. When only one child has the condition the

24

couple should be referred to a clinical geneticist to make certain that a rare autosomal recessive condition has not been missed. If more than one child is affected, then an autosomal recessive mode of inheritance should be assumed, once the doctor is certain that neither parent carries any evidence of the abnormality in a less obvious form, which would suggest a dominant condition of variable penetrance.

Acquired diseases

Iron deficiency anaemia

Iron deficiency anaemia is the commonest form of anaemia in Asian children and is of dietary origin. Maternal iron deficiency in pregnancy and prematurity and low birth weight are both important factors, as is prolonged milk feeding and the late introduction of solids. Infants who are exclusively breast fed for a year or 18 months develop severe iron deficiency anaemia. The use of artificial milks, fortified with small amounts of iron, reduces the severity of the anaemia but does not necessarily prevent it.

A vegetarian diet in Britain, as eaten by strict Hindu families, results in iron deficiency, but many Hindu parents in Britain give their children meat and eggs. The peak incidence of iron deficiency is at about 3 years, though for the reasons already discussed the condition may develop much earlier. On a vegetarian diet the best sources of iron are eggs (if these are part of the normal diet of the family), dried fruit, green vegetables, whole wheat chapatis, peas, beans, and other pulses (seeds of leguminous vegetables, which when split are known as "dahl"). If one member of a family is found to have iron deficiency anaemia the other members of the family should have haemoglobin concentrations measured and receive dietary advice from someone familiar with the diet of that particular community. Though not vegetarians, children from Bangladesh are also likely to have iron deficiency anaemia.[5] Many Asian families have now adopted a partly European diet.

Poor economic circumstances in any group may result in a deficiency in iron.

A child with iron deficiency anaemia who has been living in Asia from the age of 1 year or who has become anaemic after a visit to

25

the home country should be suspected of having hookworm disease, particularly if his or her response to treatment with iron is poor (for further discussion on hookworm disease see below).

Nutritional rickets

The main factors causing rickets in Asian children are:

(*a*) lack of adequate exposure to sunlight: this affects pre-school children and adolescent girls, particularly Moslems, who may be unwilling to uncover their arms and legs in public;

(*b*) vegetarian diets: the group most at risk are strict vegetarian Hindu families (often Gujaratis);

(*c*) the use of household cows' milk for infant feeding: this contains negligible amounts of vitamin D;

(*d*) maternal deficiency of vitamin D during pregnancy and lactation.

(*e*) a poor uptake of vitamin preparations.

Clinically, nutritional rickets is seen in newborn infants, toddlers, preschool children, and adolescents.

The newborn infant—Fetal rickets may result in rickets in newborn infants, which may be recognised by craniotabes or hypocalcaemic fits, though neither are specific to rickets alone.

Infants, toddlers, and preschool children—From the age of 6 months severe rickets may develop in a child who is solely breast fed by a mother deficient in vitamin D, or who is given cows' milk and unfortified weaning foods. The site of the deformities depends on the age at onset—for example, bowing of the forearm may develop in an infant who is able to crawl. Active rickets is not always recognised as a painful disease and can cause delay in or discourage walking in a child who was previously walking quite well.

School age children—Active rickets in school children is rare as they usually have an adequate exposure to sunlight, but previously unrecognised deformities such as bow legs or genu valgum may be detected on entry to school.

Adolescent rickets—Girls are more likely to be affected than boys. Deformities are unlikely, but limb pains and backache are common presenting symptoms. Severe adolescent rickets may produce deformity of the pelvis, a cause of obstetric difficulties later on.

Prevention of nutritional rickets

Education—In 1981 the "Stop Rickets" campaign was started jointly by the Department of Health and Social Security and Save the Children Fund to inform and educate Asian communities and health workers about the causes, prevention, and detection of nutritional rickets. In September 1984 the "Asian Mother and Baby" campaign was launched by the same organisations to improve attendance at antenatal clinics and to encourage breast feeding.

Nutrition—Each Asian group should be considered separately because their dietary customs, religious beliefs, and socioeconomic circumstances are different. Leaflets in the main Asian languages on antenatal care, nutrition, rickets, and breast feeding are available from clinics or the Health Education Council. Information about instruction material for health workers for both campaigns can be obtained from the Save the Children Fund. In practice the vitamin D content of the typical diet of most Asian families makes a very small contribution to their vitamin D intake. Mothers who are bottle feeding their babies should be advised to use one of the standard baby milks, which are all fortified with vitamin D. Baby milks should be continued, instead of cows' milk, up to the age of 1 year. Other foods that normally contain added vitamin D are baby cereals and breakfast foods. Most weaning foods containing fruit and vegetables used by Asian mothers (who are generally unwilling to use those containing meat) are now fortified, with vitamin D.

Vitamin supplements—The standard "children's vitamin drops" supplied through child health clinics and welfare food distribuion centres are cheap and available free to families claiming supplementary benefit or family income supplement for children up to the age of 5 years (for further information see DHSS leaflet MV11 November, 1983). Five drops given once daily contain 7 μg vitamin D (280 IU), 200 μg vitamin A, and 20 mg vitamin C (the daily requirement of vitamin D is 7.5 μg up to the age of 1 year and 10 μg from 1 year onwards). These vitamin drops should be given from the age of 1 month and continued up to 5 years. Older children who are considered to be especially susceptible to rickets should also be given the vitamin drops. Children should not be receiving other preparations containing vitamin D in addition to the drops as there is a risk of overdose in such circumstances.

27

Intestinal infections

The most common viral infection of the gut is due to the rotavirus, which is related to poor socioeconomic circumstances.

Bacterial infections may be acquired while visiting Asia, from an infected person within the family, or from infected food. Newborn infants can be infected during delivery if the mother is a carrier of pathogenic bacteria.

Shigellosis—In infants shigellosis may be a septicaemic illness and in those aged under 5 years the initial fever may be accompanied by a convulsion. The symptoms are a high temperature and sudden onset of severe diarrhoea with blood and mucus in the stool, but in about 25% of cases there is no visible blood.

Salmonellosis (numerous strains of non-typhoid *Salmonella* also *S typhi* and *S paratyphi* A, B, and C)—*Non-typhoid salmonellosis* causes profuse diarrhoea sometimes with streaks of blood and mucus. A septicaemic illness with splenomegaly occurs in older children and mimics tuberculous meningitis. Typhoid and parathyroid fever affect mainly schoolchildren; severe frontal headache is a common initial symptom followed by vomiting, abdominal pain, and diarrhoea. The rash is difficult to detect in dark skinned children. Infection of children in Britain from cases or carriers is not uncommon.

Intestinal protozoal infections

Giardiasis should be considered when there is chronic diarrhoea and colicky pain with pale, frothy stools and increased flatus, producing in its chronic form a condition like coeliac disease.

Amoebiasis causes diarrhoea and tenesmus with blood and mucus but is less acute than bacterial dysentery; occasionally severe intestinal haemorrhage with shock occurs. Amoebic and bacillary dysentery may occur together.

Intestinal worm infestations

Roundworm infestation (ascariasis) is extremely common in children born in the Indian subcontinent and may be acquired during a visit there. Although infants may be infested, children aged 1–5 years are the most common sufferers. The diagnosis may be determined by the passage of one or two worms from the rectum or from the nose, which may be frightening for the parents. Other symptoms may be colicky abdominal pain or actual intestinal obstruction. In heavily infested children pre-existing malnutrition may be exacerbated. The life of the adult worm is about one year. Infestation in Britain is unlikely. The diagnosis can easily be made by identifying the ova in the stool. Eosinophilia is unlikely to be observed.

Hookworm infestation (ankylostomiasis) is as common as ascariasis infestation, and the two often coexist. Infestation usually occurs in toddlers, but infants are occasionally infested. No intestinal symptoms occur, but in heavily infested children hypochromic microcytic (iron deficiency) anaemia slowly develops. The diagnosis is made by identifying ova in the stools; a test for faecal occult blood is usually positive. Infestation does not occur in Britain but if untreated infestation with ankylostoma may persist for up to four years.

Lactase deficiency

Lactase deficiency (lactose malabsorption, intolerance or maldigestion) occurs in around 70% of adults in south India, but in only 33% of the adult population of north India.[6] This does not mean that all those with low levels of intestinal lactase necessarily develop symptoms after drinking milk or milk products; for fuller discussion see under chapter 6: Chinese and Vietnamese families.

Malaria

Malaria in children born in the United Kingdom is acquired during visits to the home country. A few older children entering the country for the first time develop a relapse of malaria acquired previously. Many parents do not realise that the area from which they came, previously free from malaria, may once again have become malarious and therefore do not take any precautions on their return to Asia. Infants are rarely given antimalarial drugs in the mistaken but widespread belief that these drugs are too toxic for them; dosage of antimalarial drugs should be based on estimated surface area and the fractionated amount should be given. Malaria is never acquired in Britain (with very rare exceptions of infected mosquitoes arriving by air) and cannot be transmitted to other people in the United Kingdom.

29

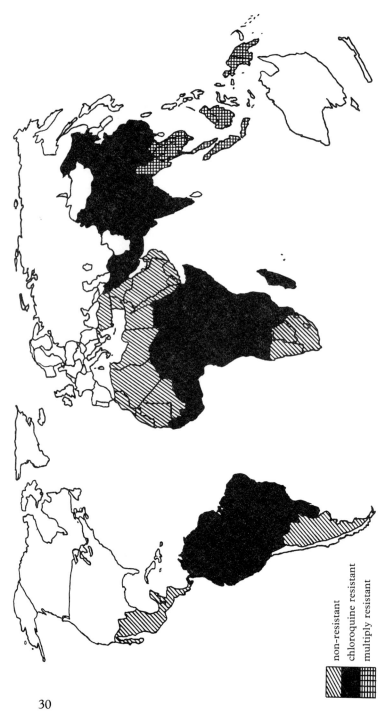

non-resistant

chloroquine resistant

multiply resistant

Areas where malaria prophylaxis is recommended (1987). Note that this map is for illustrative purposes only, and should not be used as a basis for clinical advice. Check up-to-date recommendations before prescribing (reproduced from Fuller JHS and Toon PD, Medical Practice in a

Malaria should be considered whenever fever develops suddenly in a child who has recently returned from Asia. In those aged under 5 years a febrile convulsion may occur. In a first attack the spikes of fever are often irregular and the spleen may not be palpable during the first two days after the onset of fever.

Infections acquired in the Indian subcontinent are invariably due either to *Plasmodium vivax* infection (benign tertian malaria), which produces a fairly mild disease or to *Plasmodium falciparum* infection (malignant tertian malaria), which can produce a severe and occasionally fatal illness. Falciparum malaria should be suspected when any of the following features are present.

(1) Convulsions or coma with a variable degree of fever, a meningitis-like picture, hemiplegia, or confusional state may indicate cerebral malaria. This condition is an acute emergency and should be treated with parenteral chloroquine (or quinine if there is a possibility of chloroquine resistance, which is most likely in infection acquired in Bangladesh or eastern India), but not before thick and thin blood films have been examined. All hospitals should carry supplies of parenteral chloroquine and quinine. (2) Hyperpyrexia. (3) Fever, diarrhoea, vomiting, and shock. (4) Pallor, jaundice, and splenomegaly with fever; this condition is sometimes mistaken for hepatitis A.

Recurrences of benign tertian malaria may occur up to two years after exposure and falciparum malaria up to six weeks or, exceptionally, up to one year after infection. Congenital malaria sometimes occurs in Britain, and may be due to vivax or falciparum infections. The usual age of onset is 4–6 weeks, with fever, irritability, anorexia, jaundice, and hepatosplenomegaly.

Kala azar (visceral leishmaniasis)

Kala azar is not uncommon in Bangladesh and should be considered in a chronically ill child with intermittent fever, lassitude, and a firm enlargement of the liver and spleen. The infection may have been acquired before the child came to Britain or on a visit to Asia. The incubation period is usually two to six months but may be as short as three to four weeks or as long as two years.

31

Tuberculosis

When the possibility of tuberculosis is considered the first thing to look for is a BCG scar, though this is not an absolute guarantee of protection. Primary tuberculosis should be considered in children who fail to gain weight or who lose weight for no obvious reason. A strongly positive result from a Mantoux or Heaf test invariably indicates an active infection. Respiratory tuberculosis in Asian children sometimes takes atypical forms, and the adult type of infection with cavitation may occur. Tuberculosis should also be suspected in any chronic lung condition that fails to clear up within two or three weeks.[7]

Less common forms of infection are abdominal tuberculosis, which may occur with intestinal haemorrhage, ascites, or obstruction, or bone or joint infection. Miliary and meningeal infections are fairly common.

Traditional practices and medicine

Traditionally in Asia a black eye make-up is put round the eyes and inside the lids in babies and small children, partly for its cosmetic effect and partly because it is thought to protect the eyes against infection. Originally made from soot from oil lamps and vegetable dyes or antimony sulphide, an adulterated form of surma is now made from lead sulphide;[8] cumulatively, lead can be absorbed in sufficient amounts to cause lead poisoning.[9 10] The importation into Britain of this lead-containing preparation has been banned, but some of it may still be brought into the country through non-commercial channels. Suitable hypoallergenic make-up preparations can be substituted quite safely. Kajil may also contain lead and is used in the same way as surma but is in the form of an ointment. Several medicines for infants also contain lead, which may be prescribed by practitioners of traditional Indian medicine (hakims for unani medicine and vaids for the ayurvedic system).[11]

A similar substance known as al kohl is used in Arab countries and may also contain lead.

Bizarre symptoms which cannot be related to known diseases or the side effects of prescribed drugs may be due to herbal or other medicines prescribed by "traditional" practitioners.

Some common problems

Illiteracy is not uncommon,[12] particularly in older women who have spent their childhood in the subcontinent. Leaflets and instructions in the appropriate language may therefore not meet the need, though it is unusual to find a family without at least one adolescent or school age member who is completely fluent in English. If there is a possibility of non-compliance because of language difficulties, however, and failure to take the prescribed drugs may have serious consequences, as in tuberculosis, it is essential to obtain the help of a competent interpreter. The use of children as interpreters should be discouraged, except for the most straightforward situations.

Apparent refusal to breast feed—Many Asian women believe that colostrum is harmful to the baby and may therefore be reluctant to breast feed their baby during the first two or three days. If this is the mother's belief it should be respected and it should not be assumed that she does not wish to breast feed at all.

Carriers of hepatitis B virus in pregnancy—From 3% to 10% of adults in the Indian subcontinent are potentially infective carriers of hepatitis B virus and can infect an infant at or after delivery. An infant infected at birth can become an asymptomatic carrier, who is infective for many years and may occasionally develop acute or chronic liver disease or hepatocellular carcinoma in adult life. It is therefore important to screen all pregnant Asian women at their first antenatal visit. As infection within the family is common women who have been born in Britain and have never left this country should be included in the screening programme. If the mother is found to be infective special precautions should be taken at delivery to prevent infection of the infant and medical and nursing staff. The infant should be given specific hepatitis B immunoglobulin and hepatitis B vaccine, according to the schedule described for Chinese and Vietnamese families. As the incidence of the carrier state is two to three times higher in women from south east Asia than in those from the Indian subcontinent the management of this problem will be discussed in greater detail in chapter 6: Chinese and Vietnamese Families.

Neonatal jaundice—As G6PD deficiency is not uncommon in Asian families this possibility should always be considered when non-obstructive jaundice develops on the second or third day of life. Girls may be affected (for further discussion see chapter 5: Families from the Mediterranean and Aegean), but boys are affected 40 times more often in most communities. In preterm infants or when other factors are contributing to the jaundice an exchange transfusion may be required.

Small stature, particularly in boys, is a common cause of parental anxiety among the Bengalis from Bangladesh. Generally, both parents are small but would like their children to be tall to cope with possible physical aggression. The presenting complaint is usually that "he is not growing." This may be true but is more likely to mean that the child is not as tall as the parents would like and is in fact growing at a normal rate but at or below the third centile for British children. Having excluded chronic disease and the more obvious endocrine disorders, the parents may accept that nothing can be done except to confirm a normal rate of growth by measuring the child's height again after six months; or a growth hormone stimulation test may be needed to add more convincing evidence.

Anaemia without splenomegaly—Iron deficiency is the commonest cause of moderate or severe anaemia and should be considered first; the causes of iron deficiency have already been discussed. In strictly vegetarian families folic acid or vitamin B_{12} dieficiency may occur and should be suspected initially from the appearance of the blood film. In these nutritional anaemias splenomegaly does not occur; if it is present an alternative diagnosis should be considered.

Anaemia with hepatosplenomegaly—In children who have never been to the Indian subcontinent or outside Europe the most likely diagnosis is one of the haemoglobinopathies. Homozygous β thalassaemia (thalassaemia major) is the most common condition, but haemoglobin D thalassaemia or haemoglobin E thalassaemia are also possible; sickle cell anaemia is very rare. (For discussion on geographical distribution of the haemoglobinopathies see chapter 7: Afro-Caribbean and African families.) In children who have lived in or visited the subcontinent additional diagnoses such as chronic malaria and kala azar (in India, West Bengal, Assam, and Bangladesh predominantly) may have to be considered.

Hepatitis—Chronic active hepatitis B infection or early cirrhosis is not uncommon in children presenting with chronic ill health and an enlarged liver. Splenomegaly is found only in advanced cirrhosis with portal hypertension in older children. Hepatitis A may develop in children who have recently returned from a visit to the Indian subcontinent; chronic or persistent liver disease is a rare sequel to this form of hepatitis.

1 Karan V K, Prasad S N, Prasad T B. Sickle cell disorder in aboriginal tribes in Chotanagpur. *Indian Paediat* 1978; 15:287–91.
2 Grant D B, Smith I. Survey of neonatal screening for primary hypothyroidism in England, Wales and Northern Ireland 1982–4. *Br Med J* 1988; 296:1355–8.
3 Rosenthal M, Addison G M, Price D A. Congenital hypothyroidism: increased incidence in Asian families. *Arch Dis Child* 1988; 63:790–3.
4 Darr A, Modell B. The frequency of consanguineous marriages in British Pakistanis. *J Med Genet* 1988; 25:186–90.
5 Harris R J, Armstrong D, Ali R, Loynes A. Nutritional survey of Bangladeshi children aged under 5 years in the London borough of Tower Hamlets. *Arch Dis Child* 1983; 58:428–32.
6 Tandon R K, Joshi Y K, Singh D S, Natendranathan M, Balakrishnan V, Lal K. Lactose intolerance in North and South Indians. *Am J Clin Nutr* 1981; 34:943–6.
7 Darbyshire J H. We don't have tuberculosis in this country any more . . . do we? *Maternal and Child Health* 1978; 8:176–82.
8 Green S D R, Lealman G T, Aslam M, Davis S S. Surma and blood lead concentrations. *Public Health* 1979; 93:371–6.
9 Warley M A, Blackledge P, O'Gorman P. Lead poisoning from eye cosmetics. *Br Med J* 1968; i:117.
10 Fernando N P, Healy M A, Aslam M, Davis S S, Hussein A. Lead poisoning and traditional practices: consequences for world health. A study in Kuwait. *Public Health* 1981; 95:250–60.
11 Aslam M, Healy M. Present and future trends in the health care of British-Asian children. *Nursing Times* 1982; 78:1353–4.
12 Aslam M, Davis S S, Fletcher R. Compliance in medication by Asian immigrants. *Nursing Times* 1979; 75:931–2.

Further reading

Arthurton M. Immigrant children and the day-to-day work of a paediatrician. *Arch Dis Child* 1972; 47:126–30.

5 Families from the Mediterranean and Aegean

Greek Cypriots and Greeks

The groups of major importance, roughly in order of the size of their communities in the United Kingdom are: Greek Cypriots, Turkish Cypriots, Greeks, Italians, and Turkish families from the mainland.

Both Greek Cypriots and Greeks have been in Britain for many years, mainly in our large cities. Greek Cypriots originally came to London in small numbers in the 1920s, but much larger immigrations occurred in 1950–60 and again in 1974. In London the Greek community originally settled in Soho and the Cypriots in Camden Town. The main areas in London where Greek Cypriots now live are: Camden, Hackney, Haringey, and Islington; Greek families are mainly in north London. There are Greek and Greek Cypriot communities in most of the large cities in Britain. Members of both communities are largely employed in the clothing trade, in restaurants and groceries, and in other service industries.

Religion—The Greek Orthodox Church, to which both communities belong, has not raised any moral or ethical difficulties about fetal diagnosis or termination of pregnancy in relation to β thalassaemia (for further discussion on genetically determined diseases see below).

Language—Greek is usually spoken at home, with English as the second language. There are rarely serious language difficulties at entry to school.

Naming system—In Greek Cypriots the wife takes the husband's surname, and the children take the father's first name as their surname. In Britain, however, children increasingly taken their father's surname, thus conforming to British practice. Greek

36

women may retain their maiden name after marriage or put their unmarried surname before their husband's surname; the children may use their mother's "surname" as theirs or use their father's surname. With Cypriot families it is most important to find out whether the family comes from the Turkish or the Greek part of Cyprus. Some idea may be obtained from the religion recorded in their notes: Greek Cypriots may be recorded as Christians or as belonging to the Greek Orthodox church, while Turkish Cypriots are Moslems. Some indication may be obtained from the names. Common Greek or Greek Cypriot boys' names are: Antonis, Christos, Petros, Savvas, and girls names: Eleni, Maria, Niki. Many Greek or Greek Cypriot surnames end in *ou* (Georgiou), meaning "son of", or in *aides* (Nicolaides).

Genetically determined diseases

β Thalassaemia (Mediterranean anaemia, Cooley's anaemia)

β Thalassaemia, inherited as an autosomal recessive disease, occurs in both communities but is more common among the Cypriots. In the homozygous state (thalassaemia major) there is an inability to make adult haemoglobin (HbA). Heterozygotes (thalassaemia minor, thalassaemia trait) are invariably asymptomatic but can be reliably detected by screening. In north London Modell has shown that about 17% of the Cypriot (Greek and Turkish) community have thalassaemia minor and 3% of marriages have a one in four risk of producing a child with thalassaemia major;[1] without intervention about one in every 120 live births within this community would be expected to result in an affected child; the birth of a baby with homozygous β thalassaemia is now quite rare in the Greek and Cypriot communities in London.

Clinically, thalassaemia major usually presents between the ages of 6 months and 1 year with pallor, listlessness, and failure to thrive; severe anaemia occurs, often with a haemoglobin concentration as low as 3–5 g/dl, and abdominal distension due to hepatosplenomegaly. Older children, if untreated or undertreated, may develop the so called "Mongolian" facial appearance due to expansion of the frontal and maxillary bones. Blood films show red cells of irregular shape and size, with numerous target cells. On electrophoresis there is a high concentration of fetal haemoglobin

37

(HbF) and an almost complete absence of HbA; concentrations of HbA$_2$ are normal or slightly raised and are of no diagnostic importance. Children with suspected thalassaemia major should be admitted to hospital immediately for confirmation of the diagnosis and transfusion. They should be looked after at a special clinic or by a paediatrician or haematologist with a particular interest in the condition. Treatment consists of regular blood transfusions and injections or infusions with desferrioxamine to reduce the overload of iron or marrow transplant.

Though thalassaemia minor is of no clinical importance, its detection is important in preventing thalassaemia major. The characteristic microcytosis of thalassaemia minor can be detected by a Coulter counter and confirmed by a high concentration of HbA$_2$. With the support of a well informed and enthusiastic community the incidence of thalassaemia major in north London has been reduced by 60% over the past seven years. All Greek and Cypriot women (and also in practice all women of "non-British" origin are included) are screened at their first attendance at the antenatal clinic; the husbands of women with thalassaemia minor are then also tested. Couples who are both heterozygous are offered fetal diagnosis by chorionic villus biopsy at 10–14 weeks of pregnancy, and termination if a homozygous fetus is found. Obviously, with a community that is well informed about thalassaemia screening should be extended to school leavers, but this would need to be supported by a programme of education on the implications of having thalassaemia minor.

The family doctor and β thalassaemia—The possibility of thalassaemia major should be considered in young children with severe anaemia whose families have originated from Mediterranean or Aegean countries or Bulgaria, Soviet Central Asia,[2] or the Indian subcontinent and south east Asia. The figure shows the world distribution of β thalassaemia. Treatment of a child with thalassaemia creates an emotional and often economic strain on the family, who require support from their family doctor and the community services. Treatment with iron or other haematinics should not be given unless requested by a specialist clinic; folic acid is not required if the child is on a programme of regular transfusions. Parents or adolescents requesting screening, and the families of all patients with thalassaemia major and minor, should be referred to the nearest appropriate haematology department (see Useful

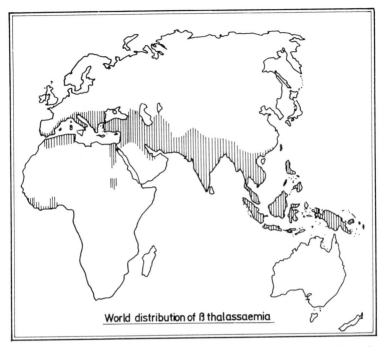

World distribution of β thalassaemia. Reproduced from Thalassaemia Syndromes. *3rd ed. Weatherall D J, Clegg J B. Oxford: Blackwell Scientific Publications, 1981, with permission of authors and publishers.*

addresses for centres in London). Families or individuals requiring further advice should be referred to the United Kingdom Thalassaemia Society (see Useful addresses).

Glucose-6-phosphate dehydrogenase (G6PD) deficiency

G6PD deficiency is transmitted through an X-linked intermediate gene with variable expression in the heterozygous female (see below); the affected person has a notable reduction of the enzyme G6PD in the red cells, causing rapid haemolysis in response to several drugs (table I) and also during acute infections, particularly hepatitis, and in diabetic ketoacidosis. Neonatal jaundice is also a common problem. Three main variants of this condition occur: the Mediterranean, the African, and the Far Eastern forms. In the

39

TABLE I—*Drugs likely to cause haemolysis in G6PD deficiency**

Antimalarials	Primaquine
	Pamaquin
	Pentaquine
Sulphonamides	Sulphanilamide
	Sulphacetamide
	Sulphapyridine
	Sulphamethoxazole (in Bactrim and Septrin)
	Silver sulphadiazine (surface application for burns)
Sulphones	Dapsone (in Maloprim, prophylaxis for malaria)
	Thiazosulphone
Nitrofurans	Nitrofurantoin (Furadantin)
Analgesics	Acetanilide
Miscellaneous	Methylene blue
	Nalidixic acid (Negram)
	Naphthalene
	Niridazole
	Phenylhydrazine
	Toluidine blue
	Trinitrotoluene

Table modified from: Wintrobe M M, Lee G R, Boggs D R, *et al. Clinical Hematology*. 8th ed. Philadelphia: Lea and Febiger, 1981:792, with permission from authors and publishers.

*Different authors give slightly different lists of drugs.

Mediterranean and Far Eastern forms, but not in the African, contact with the broad bean (*Vicia faba*) produces a particularly severe haemolysis (favism); even sniffing the pollen may be enough to cause a haemolytic crisis. Table II summarises the main differences between the three types of G6PD deficiency.

Haemolytic crises—As would be expected males are more often affected, but in all three types the gene is so common that homozygous females, having received the gene on the X chromosome from each parent, are not uncommon. Homozygous females are usually as severely affected as males, while heterozygous females may be mildly affected. The haemolysis is so rapid that severe anaemia, often down to a haemoglobin concentration of 3–4 g/dl, develops before any jaundice becomes obvious. Haemoglobin should be looked for in the urine as evidence of haemolysis. The patient requires immediate admission to hospital for transfusion. Confirmation of the diagnosis may have to wait until the disappearance of transfused cells and the maturation of the young cells produced by the patient in response to haemolysis. The diagnosis can, however, usually be inferred by investigating the parents and siblings.

Neonatal jaundice—In some enzyme deficient infants neonatal hyperbilirubinaemia occurs without any drug contact. Jaundice usually develops on the second or third day, reaching a peak around the fourth to fifth day. Exchange transfusion may be required, particularly in preterm infants or when there are other factors causing hyperbilirubinaemia. The possibility of G6PD deficiency should be considered in infants of either sex with "non-British" parents or mothers (G6PD deficiency, apparently of the Mediterranean type, is not uncommon in the Indian sub-continent). It is rare for parents to be aware of the disease in their family. When the diagnosis has been confirmed in the child the rest of the family should be investigated and the clinical and genetic implications fully explained. Affected people and their family doctor should be given a list of the drugs that must be avoided (table I).

Lactase deficiency

Lactase deficiency (lactose malabsorption, intolerance, or maldigestion) is present in about 40% of adults in Greece[3] and there is probably a similar proportion in Greek Cypriots in Britain. Only a small fraction of such lactase deficient adults or older children (over 6 years) develop symptoms after drinking milk or milk

TABLE II—*The variants of G6PD deficiency*

	Mediterranean and Far Eastern*	African (including Afro-Caribbeans)
Enzyme activity as normal (%)	0–5%	5–15%
Latent period after exposure (hours)	3–24	24–36
Haemoglobinuria	Always	Common
Anaemia	Haemoglobin often <6 g/dl	Haemoglobin rarely <6 g/dl
Duration of haemolysis	Continuous if drug is continued; sometimes fatal	Self limiting even if drug is continued (not advised); rarely fatal
Favism	Yes	No
Neonatal hyperbilirubinaemia	Common, without drug contact	Without drug contact, in preterm and term infants
Affected females	Common	Common

*Though genetically distinct the Mediterranean and Far Eastern variants behave in a similar manner.

41

products. For a fuller discussion see chapter 6: Chinese and Vietnamese families.

Turkish and Turkish Cypriot families

A few Turkish Cypriots came to Britain in the 1920s, but many more arrived in 1947–50 and again in 1960–2. In London they have settled mainly in the north (Haringey, Islington, Stoke Newington), the east (Hackney), and the south east (Bromley, Catford, Lewisham, New Cross). There are smaller communities in most of the larger cities. Turkish families came to Britain more recently and have tended to settle in the same areas as the Cypriots. Members of both communities work in the clothing industry, in groceries and restaurants, and in other service industries.

Religion—Both communities are Moslem, though with usually less strict observance than in groups from the Middle East and Pakistan or Bangladesh. There is an absolute prohibition on eating pork or pork products but less insistence on halal meat. Marriage is monogamous (by law in Turkey). Problems about necropsies are rare, but the parents should be approached with gentleness and tact. Parents should also be consulted about preference for a woman doctor if their daughter has to be examined at the surgery or outpatient clinic.

Language—Turkish is spoken at home by both groups, but Turkish parents may have no second language, except possibly German if they have worked in West Germany. Learning English presents difficulties for Turkish adults, and an interpreter may be required. Pronunciation of Turkish names is not as difficult as it may appear, as it is largely phonetic and each letter is pronounced (there are no double consonant sounds as in the English "th"), apart from ğ, which only lengthens the preceding vowel and is not sounded: c is like j; ç is pronounced "ch" as in church; ş is "sh" as in shoe; ö and ü are as in the German; i is the English e as in meat; ı is as in "were" or "Sir"; and g is hard as in "get".

Naming system—The naming system is usually the same for Turkish and Turkish Cypriot families, but it is impossible to generalise. The wife and children usually take the father's first name as their surname. Many families, however, have adopted the British system and take the father's family name (surname) as their own. It is essential to find out which system the family is using. Typical boys' names are: Gültekin, Mehmet, Suleyman, Turgay, Yusuf, and girls' names: Ayşe, Gulay, Hatije, or they may be the same as a boy's name but with a terminal e as in Ermin(e). The ending *oğlu* means "son of."

Medical conditions found in the children—β thalassaemia and G6PD deficiency occur in both groups with a higher incidence in Turkish Cypriots, though it is probably not as high as that in Greek Cypriots. The incidence of lactase deficiency is probably similar in the Turkish population to that in Greece.[3] There are no other conditions specific to these two communities.

Italian families

Italian families, originally mainly in the catering trade, have been in Britain for many generations; some immigration occurred in the Luton and Bedford areas after the end of the second world war, and there has been further immigration into larger cities since then.

Religion—Most Italians are Roman Catholics with a strong religious objection to termination of pregnancy, so fetal diagnosis is pointless. Nevertheless, and particularly in relation to β thalassaemia, it should not be assumed without discussion that all parents will have these views.

Language—Italian is normally spoken at home with English as a second language. There are rarely any serious language difficulties at entry to school.

Medical conditions found in the children—Both β thalassaemia and G6PD deficiency occur quite commonly, particularly in families originating from southern Italy, Sardinia, and Sicily. Lactase deficiency is present in about 56–70% of adults and older children. There is evidence[4] that this condition is responsible for recurrent abdominal pain in some Italian children aged over the age of 6–7 years.

1 Modell B. Prevention of the haemoglobinopathies. *Br Med Bull* 1983; **39**:386–91.
2 Weatherall D J, Clegg J B. *Thalassaemia syndromes*. 3rd ed. Oxford: Blackwell Scientific, 1981; 299–300.
3 Scrimshaw N S, Murray E B. The acceptability of milk and milk products in populations with a high incidence of lactose intolerance. *Am J Clin Nutr* 1988; 48 Suppl:1083–1159.

4 Ceriani R, Zuccato E, Fontana M, *et al.* Lactose malabsorbtion and recurrent abdominal pain in Italian children. *J Pediatr Gastroenterol Nutr* 1988; 7:852–7.

Useful addresses

Thalassaemia Society UK, 107 Nightingale Lane, London N8 (01 348 0437/2553)

George Marsh Sickle Cell and Thalassaemia Centre, St Ann's Hospital, St Ann's Road, London N15 3TH (01 800 0121 ext 4230, or 809-1797

Cypriot (Greek) Advisory Service, 26 Crowndale Road, London NW1 1TT (01 388 7971)

Cyprus Turkish Association, 34 D'Arblay Street, London W1A 4YL (01 437 4940)

For addresses of centres where advice and counselling on thalassaemia are provided, apply to one of the above addresses.

6 Chinese and Vietnamese families

Chinese families

For many generations there have been Chinese communities in our major ports, but only during the past 20 years have greater numbers come to Britain, mainly from Hong Kong, Malaysia, and Singapore. In London most Chinese families live in Camden, Islington, Lambeth, and the City of Westminster, though there are smaller communities or single families scattered all over London, owing to the large number of Chinese restaurants. In the rest of Britain the pattern is similar, with large communities in Liverpool, Manchester, and Bristol. There are also a few families from the People's Republic of China in London, mainly attached to or working in the Chinese Embassy. The ethnic Chinese families who came to the United Kingdom from Vietnam have rather different problems and are considered later.

Social structure and family life

Perhaps more than any other immigrant group the Chinese have tended to retain their social structure and cultural attitudes with little contact with local or national activities. The extended family is a very important aspect of their social life; for the children, respect for parents, relatives, older people, and "authority figures" such as teachers is an essential part of their attitude to life.

Religion—There are many Buddhists and also Christians of various denominations. So called "ancestor worship," more properly reverence or respect for one's ancestors, is important to most Chinese families and means looking to their ancestors for guidance. It is a way of life not a religion, and its practice is quite compatible with membership of a formal religious group. In the

45

People's Republic of China there is no formal religion; religious worship is tolerated but not encouraged.

Language—Families from urban Hong Kong usually speak Cantonese while those from the New Territories may speak Hakka or Cantonese, or both. Many families from Malaysia and Singapore speak Hokien. Mandarin is also widely understood. Written Chinese, being in the form of ideographs, is, of course, understood by all Chinese people.

Naming system—The Chinese normally put the family name (surname) first, followed by the given names. In Britain, however, many families have adopted the British system, with the family name last, so it is essential to clear up this point at the beginning. When asking someone's name it is best to say, "What is your family name?" and "What is your personal or given name?" Older women may have retained their maiden names after marriage without adding the husband's family name, but this is becoming less common. When a whole family is registered, as in general practice, and the wife is using her maiden name it is best to put in brackets (wife of Mr . . .). Children normally take the father's family name; they may have both English and Chinese names, or for use in school they may use an English translation of their Chinese given names. Thus "Beautiful Morning" in Chinese becomes, more prosaically, "Dawn" in English.

General medical problems

Chinese families do not use medical or social and community services as much as do British families. Parents may be reluctant to go to a doctor or hospital if they cannot explain what is wrong or are worried that they may not understand the instructions about treatment or drugs that have been prescribed. Similar fears and traditional self-sufficiency may prevent them from claiming the social benefits to which they are entitled, resulting sometimes in avoidable hardship or ill health.

Many families consult Chinese practitioners of traditional medicine or buy herbal remedies before resorting to Western medicine, though they are more likely to take an ill child straight to their doctor or to hospital.

Blood tests—There is often reluctance, or even refusal, to have blood taken for investigations, on the ground that removal of blood causes weakness. Understandably, there may be considerable resistance if many or repeated blood samples are requested.

Diet—There may be conflict between the dietary advice given by an antenatal clinic and the traditional changes in diet that are determined by the concept of "heating" and "cooling" foods. As pregnancy is regarded as a "hot" condition the mother may reduce her intake of "hot" foods such as red meat, oils, or fatty dishes. Dietary adjustments during pregnancy may require much time and discussion. A child may find food provided by hospitals unacceptable, and the parents should be allowed to bring food into the ward. Weaning may also cause difficulties; most Chinese infants are weaned on to congee (rice porridge) mixed with chopped meat and vegetables, and the mother may not accept the advice given by the health visitor or advisors at a baby clinic. Adequate supplements of vitamin D are important. Older children and adults do not drink milk, and it is pointless to try to force them to take it as it may cause abdominal discomfort or diarrhoea (for further discussion see below under lactase deficiency).

Hepatitis B

Hepatitis B (HBV infection) carriers in pregnancy[1]—About 10–20% of adults in south east Asia are potentially infective carriers of hepatitis B; most are asymptomatic, but a few have evidence of hepatic disease (see below). In sub-Saharan Africa, the Indian subcontinent, and the Mediterranean area about 3–10% are carriers. Apart from special categories (see below), the indigenous population of the United Kingdom and the Afro-Caribbean community are very rarely carriers. As infection occurs within family groups women belonging to the ethnic groups mentioned above who have been born and remained in Britain all their lives may be infective. Pregnant women in all the at risk groups should, therefore, be screened at their first antenatal visit. In addition, irrespective of ethnic or geographical considerations, other groups who should be screened are: (*a*) women who have had hepatitis B during the last trimester of pregnancy; (*b*) women who have received numerous blood transfusions for β thalassaemia major, sickle cell anaemia, or other haemoglobinopathies; and (*c*) those known for or suspected of drug abuse by self injection. Those whose blood contains

47

hepatitis surface antigen (HBsAg) should be screened by hepatitis B virus DNA analysis, which is the most sensitive indicator of infectivity. Women with HBsAg, particularly those who also have HBeAg, can infect their infants around the time of delivery, or subsequently. Infants infected at birth (transplacental infection is rare) commonly become asymptomatic carriers without adverse effects during early life and are major contributors to the pool of persistent carriers in the community. Rarely, such children may develop clinical hepatic diseases (see below). Infants or children infected some time after birth are less likely to become persistent carriers.

Management of pregnancy and delivery—All pregnant women in the groups at risk mentioned above should be screened at their first antenatal visit. If the mother is found to be a carrier all blood samples should be treated as infectious, according to the standard procedure for hepatitis B. During delivery special precautions should be taken to prevent infection of those conducting the delivery, and maternal blood, placenta, and membranes should be regarded as infective.

Management of the newborn infant—All maternal blood should be cleaned off the infant's skin, and the stomach should be aspirated to remove swallowed maternal blood. The following procedure is recommended; as soon after birth as possible, and in any case within 48 hours of delivery 200 mg (200 IU, 0·5 ml) of specific hepatitis B immunoglobulin should be given intramuscularly, and at the same time 10 mg (0·5 ml) of hepatitis B vaccine should be given intramuscularly, at a different site. A second dose of vaccine is given one month later and a third dose six months after the first. The immunoglobulin should be obtained from the Central Public Health Laboratory, Hepatitis Epidemiology Unit, Colindale, London, NW9 5HT, tel: 01 205 7041, which should be consulted in difficult or doubtful cases.

Liver disease in childhood—In infancy and childhood hepatitis B infection can cause various responses, ranging from the asymptomatic production of antibodies, with or without the carrier state, to acute hepatitis, chronic hepatitis, cirrhosis, or hepatocellular carcinoma in adult life. A manifestation that is unique to childhood is acute hepatitis with papular acrodermatitis (Gianotti-Crosti syndrome).

Conditions found in the children

Genetically determined conditions

Haemoglobin Barts hydrops fetalis (also known as *a* thalassaemia hydrops) occurs when the infant is homozygous for a type of *a* thalassaemia, which is asymptomatic in its heterozygous form. It is common throughout south east Asia and in the south of China, but its distribution in the rest of the People's Republic of China is not yet known. There is an increased incidence of toxaemia in the mother, and the pregnancy may last for 30–40 weeks. There may be a history of stillbirths or early neonatal deaths of hydropic infants. The infant may die in utero or a few hours after delivery; despite generalised oedema the birth weight is lower than normal for the gestational age. The placenta is enlarged and oedematous and the infant anaemic, with a haemoglobin concentration of 6–7 g/dl or less. There is gross hepatosplenomegaly with the liver slightly more enlarged than the spleen. Though an anaemic hydropic infant with parents of Far Eastern origin is likely to have Hb Barts disease, it is essential to confirm the diagnosis by examining the baby's blood as diagnosis of the carrier state in the parents is difficult. On electrophoresis, the infant's blood consists mainly of Hb Barts; HbF and HbA are completely absent. No treatment is possible as these infants cannot manufacture a haemoglobin that is capable of delivering oxygen to the tissues. Genetic advice is important as there is a 1:4 chance of having a similarly affected child. Antenatal diagnosis may be practicable in the future.

Haemoglobin H disease—This form of *a* thalassaemia results from a doubly heterozygous state for two different *a* thalassaemia genes. The condition becomes obvious during the first year of life with symptoms, facial appearance, and physical signs similar to those of *β* thalassaemia major, though there is a much greater variation in the haemoglobin concentration, which is usually 7–8 g/dl. In general, the condition is less severe than *β* thalassaemia and life expectancy is reasonably good. Blood films also resemble those in thalassaemia major, but after the red cells have been incubated with cresyl blue inclusion bodies can be seen. The HbH concentration is 2–4g/dl. The chronic haemolysis that already exists may increase during acute infections or after exposure to the same drugs or conditions that cause haemolysis in G6PD deficiency (see

49

chapters on Afro-Caribbean families and Mediterranean and Aegean families). Confirmation of the heterozygous state in the parents may be extremely difficult.

β *Thalassaemia* is not uncommon in Chinese families;[2] the clinical presentation and diagnostic features have already been described.

Glucose 6 phosphate dehydrogenase deficiency—The Far Eastern form of G6PD deficiency is common in Chinese families from Hong Kong and south China, particularly Guangdong (Canton) province. The Hakka community, some members of which emigrated from Hong Kong, also has a high incidence. Though five variants of Far Eastern G6PD deficiency have been recognised, the clinical behaviour of each variant is much the same, and all are inherited through an X-linked intermediate gene with varying expression in heterozygous women, who are usually asymptomatic. Owing to the high incidence of the gene in affected groups, homozygous women are not uncommon and may be as severely affected as men. The behaviour of the Far Eastern forms of G6PD deficiency in relation to drugs, infections, the broad bean (probably) and neonatal jaundice is similar to that of the Mediterranean variant see chapter 5: Families from the Mediterranean and Aegean. Exchange transfusions for hyperbilirubinaemia in the neonatal period may be required in the absence of exposure to drugs.

Lactase deficiency (lactose intolerance, malabsorbtion, maldigestion)—For comprehensive review see Scrimshaw and Murray.[3]

It is now recognised that in most of the world's population the intestinal lactase which is present at birth declines to quite low levels in early childhood (6–7 years or earlier)[3] and remains unchanged for the rest of adult life. An increase in lactase activity cannot be induced nor can the decline be prevented by the continued consumption of milk or milk products.

About 80% of the population of northern, central, and western Europe and their descendants elsewhere, and a few nomadic tribes[4] whose survival depends upon the consumption of large amounts of goats' milk or camels' milk, retain an undiminished level of intestinal lactase throughout life. It appears that this post infancy type of lactase deficiency is inherited as an autosomal recessive trait and that lactase retention is due to a dominant gene with high penetrance.[3] The incidence of lactase deficiency in different parts of the world varies according to ethnic origin and mixing. In India about 33% of the population in the north are lactase deficient compared with 60–70% in the south.[5] The population of Italy and Greece have an intermediate incidence of deficiency.[3] Scattered published reports suggests that the Japanese, Thais, Koreans, and people of Chinese descent in Australia, America, and elsewhere have one of the highest incidences of deficiency (75–100%); these groups also have a higher incidence (60–70%)[3] of awareness of milk intolerance than other deficient groups. It therefore seems appropriate to discuss this rather confusing subject in this chapter.

There is no doubt that in a few lactase deficient children recurrent abdominal pain can be relieved by a low lactose diet;[3] confusion with milk allergy must, of course, be avoided. There seems to be no connection between lactase deficiency and the irritable bowel syndrome.[3] Evidence from numerous studies[3] suggests that the proportion of adults who become symptomatic after drinking a reasonable amount of milk (240 ml) is probably not more than 30%, and even in these subjects symptoms may not develop if the milk is taken in divided amounts or with a meal. The usual symptoms in adults and older children are abdominal distension, flatulence, abdominal pain or discomfort, and occasionally diarrhoea. Much of the confusion about the frequency of symptoms in lactase deficiency has arisen from the assumption that the incidence of symptoms due to the consumption of milk on a day to day basis is the same as that produced by the oral lactose tolerance test, which uses unphysiological amounts of lactose.

The amount of lactose is much reduced during the process of cheese-making;[3] but in some processed cheeses the lactose is put back. During the production of yoghurt the lactose is also reduced, and lactase derived from the bacteria responsible for fermentation may be liberated in the small intestine and may help in the digestion of the remaining lactose.[6] There is no evidence that the absorbtion of other nutrients is interfered with when a lactase deficient individual ingests milk,[3] or that milk or milk products are harmful in treating malnutrition in a lactase deficient population.

Acquired disease

Helminthiasis—Roundworm (*Ascaris lumbricoides*) and, less commonly, hookworm (*Ankylostoma duodenale*) may be acquired during a visit to south east Asia.

51

Emotional problems

Chinese children born in Britain usually have few language problems when they start school, particularly if the school is used to making special arrangements for children speaking little or no English. In schools where there are few non-British children, however, special facilities may not exist. Children who have come at a later age to the United Kingdom, often at 8–9 years, have great difficulties in adjustment after spending their early childhood with grandparents in Hong Kong or elsewhere. Not only do they not know their own parents and any siblings who have been born in this country, but their knowledge of English may be poor and their academic achievements quite different from those of British children of the same age. It is not always appreciated that many families from Hong Kong come from the New Territories, where the parents have had small farms, and the standard of schooling and general life is much less sophisticated than in urban Hong Kong and Kowloon.

Children with problems at school or conflicts arising from various circumstances may present to the family doctor with apparent somatic diseases, such as headache, recurrent attacks of vomiting, or abdominal pain. Chinese parents expect the school to provide homework from an early age, and at the same time the children accept their duty to help in the restaurant or shop on returning from school, which results in sleepiness at school and poor progress. Cultural conflicts may arise when a child, particularly a girl, unsuccessfully attempts to reconcile her life as an English schoolgirl during the day with being a dutiful daughter at home. Extreme forms of rejection of one or other culture may result in elective mutism at school or a refusal to talk Chinese at home. Playing truant may result from intolerable pressures at school or from racist taunting or bullying.

Vietnamese families

Since 1975 about 16 000 people from Vietnam have come to Britain. The first small group, who came in 1975, were from South Vietnam and were mostly ethnic Vietnamese. The second, much larger, group came during 1977–9, with a peak in 1979, from both

North and South Vietnam and were predominantly ethnic Chinese (80%). Of these 16 000 refugees, about 11 000 came from North Vietnam via Hong Kong, the so called "boat people." During the war, and due to the difficulties of their escape, many families were split up, and it has only recently become possible for families in Britain to apply for exit facilities for relatives who were left behind in Vietnam.

On arrival in Britain the families were housed in camps; they were then dispersed throughout Britain in single families or small groups, according to the willingness and ability of local authorities to make housing available. Whatever the reason for this policy, it caused great hardship and distress for people who, in most cases, had had no contact with the Western way of life and generally spoke no English. The result was a complete lack of integration, difficulty in helping the scattered families and in organising classes in English, and very high unemployment. They became depressed and discouraged. Recently, many families have moved to the big cities, especially London. Obviously, integration is easier for the ethnic Chinese who usually speak Cantonese; the ethnic Vietnamese may have greater difficulty in integrating. Families from Vietnam live mainly in London (south east), Birmingham, Coventry, Manchester, Wales, and in the north of Scotland.

Language—The ethnic Chinese speak Cantonese or Vietnamese, or both; ethnic Vietnamese speak Vietnamese. The Roman alphabet is in general use in Vietnam, though many of the Chinese also understand written Chinese.

Naming system—Normally, the first name is the family name or surname; this is followed by the middle name and finally the personal name. Children take their father's family name, but a woman usually keeps her maiden name after marriage without adding the husband's family name. Some families have revised the order, however, putting the surname last, to fit in with the British convention, so it is necessary to ask about this. The receptionist, nurse, or doctor should always ask how the patient would like to be addressed and should make a note of a phonetic rendering of the name below the official record, as the spelling gives little guide to pronunciation. If a name is wrongly pronounced the patient will not recognise it when it is called out.

General medical problems

Traditional medicines and methods of treatment—Many families, particularly from North Vietnam, have had little or no contact with Western medicine and have a correspondingly firm belief in traditional practitioners and methods of treatment. "Coin rubbing" produces linear ecchymoses, usually on the back; these lesions can be mistaken for non-accidental injury, with disastrous consequences. Another form of physical treatment (for persistent cough) is to pinch or squeeze the area on either side of the trachea; this is repeated down the upper part of the anterior chest wall. The bruising that results is considerable and may be puzzling if its origin is not recognised.[7]

Pregnancy and termination of pregnancy—Termination of pregnancy is accepted in Vietnam, but generally knowledge about contraception is small.

Diet—As for Chinese families.

Death—If a member of the family dies in hospital the family should be consulted about its wishes. Families from North Vietnam in particular may be reluctant to agree to a necropsy.

Conditions found in the children

Blood disorders—β thalassaemia, Hb Barts hydrops fetalis (homozygous α thalassaemia), Hb H disease, and G6PD deficiency all occur in Vietnamese families; these conditions have already been described under Chinese families.

Lactase deficiency—As for Chinese families.

Helminthiasis—Roundworm (*Ascaris lumbricoides*) infestation was particularly common in children when they arrived in Britain but should have been eradicated by now. New arrivals should, however, have their stools examined for ova and other pathogens.

Tuberculosis was also common when refugees first arrived in the United Kingdom. Most children who were tuberculin negative were given a BCG injection; some, however, may not have received it. Newly arrived children should undergo chest radiography, tuberculin testing, and BCG vaccination if they are tuberculin negative.

Hepatitis B—As for Chinese families.

1 Zuckerman A J. Perinatal transmission of hepatitis B. *Arch Dis Child* 1984; **59**:1007–9.
2 Wong H B. Haemoglobinopathies in Singapore. *J Singapore Paediatr Soc* 1967; **9**:1–27.
3 Scrimshaw N S, Murray E B. The acceptability of milk and milk products in populations with a high incidence of lactose intolerance. *Am J Clin Nutr* 1988; **48** (suppl):1083–1159.
4 Bayoumi R A L, Flatz S D, Kuhnau W, Flatz W. Beja and Nilotes: nomadic pastoralist groups in the Sudan with opposite distributions of the adult lactase phenotype. *Am J Phys Anthropol* 1982; **58**:173–8.
5 Tandou R K, Joshi Y K, Singh D S, Narendranathan M, Balakrishnan V, Lal K. Lactose intolerance in North and South Indians. *Am J Clin Nutr* 1981; **34**:943–6.
6 Kolars J C, Levitt M D, Aouji M, Savaiano D A. Yogurt: an autodigesting source of lactase. *N Engl J Med* 1984; **310**:1–3.
7 Phillips S. Bizarre physical signs and traditional Vietnamese folk medicine. *Maternal and Child Health* 1981; **6**:145–7.

Further reading

Ball R, ed. *Report of the Second National Conference on Chinese Children in Britain.* Huddersfield: National Children's Centre, 1978.
Hunt W. Chinese children in Britain: a report. *China Now* 1984; **No 110**:25–7.
Lynn I L. *The Chinese community in Liverpool.* Liverpool: Department of Sociology, University of Liverpool, 1982.
Mares P. *The Vietnamese in Britain: a handbook for health workers.* Cambridge: Cambridge Health Education Council and the National Extension College, 1982.
Pearson R. Understanding the Vietnamese in Britain. *Health Visitor Journal* 1982; **55**:426–30, 477–82, and 533–8.
Weatherall D J, Clegg J B. *Thalassaemia syndromes.* 3rd ed. Oxford: Blackwell Scientific Publications, 1981.

Useful addresses

For Chinese families:
Chinese Community Centre, 44 Gerrard Street, London W1V 7LP (01 439 3822)

Merseyside Chinese Centre, 32a Berry Street, Liverpool L1 45Q

The Pagoda of Hundred Harmony, Chinese Community Centre, Henry Street, Liverpool L1 5BU   (051 708 8833)

For Vietnamese families:
Refugee Action (Head Office), The Offices, The Cedars, Oakwood, Derby DE2 4FY   (0332 833310)

Refugee Action (London only), 240a Clapham Road, London SW9
                                        (01 735 5361)

7 Afro-Caribbean and African families

Afro-Caribbean families

The term Afro-Caribbean is now commonly used to indicate people from the West Indies who are of African origin. The population of the West Indies, however, includes many other races of which those of Indian origin are the most numerous; but most families in Britain from the West Indies are of African origin.

Afro-Caribbeans and Africans have in common three important genetically determined conditions: sickle cell disease, haemoglobin C (or more commonly the combined condition HbSC disease), and glucose 6 phosphate dehydrogenase (G6PD) deficiency. Their family structures and social problems are, however, quite different.

Immigration from the West Indies occurred mainly during the 1950s and 1960s due to a combination of economic depression in the Caribbean and vacancies in lower paid jobs in Britain. About 60% of the immigrants came from Jamaica, the remainder from Trinidad, Barbados, and the smaller islands. The main areas of settlement were London, Manchester, Leeds, Nottingham, Bristol, Northampton, and Reading.[1,2] In Reading most families came from Barbados,[2] while High Wycombe has a mainly Vincentian settlement.[2] In some cases the younger children remained at home for months or years before joining their parents in Britain. Many families retain strong ties with their homeland, and the older people regard themselves as primarily Jamaicans, Barbadians, etc, whereas those born in Britain consider themselves to be British but are conscious of their roots in the West Indies. The question "Where do you come from?" should be rephrased as, "Where does your family come from?"

Social structure and family life

Traditionally, Afro-Caribbean society is matriarchal, with the father playing an inconspicuous part. Children are looked after by the women of the extended family. When this tradition was brought to Britain several difficulties arose. Unmarried mothers had to work and, in the absence of other female members of the family, were forced to send their infants and preschool children to baby minders, who were often unregistered and gave the children little stimulation or affection. On starting school the children suffered disadvantages in language, and, later, in verbal and non-verbal reasoning and reading skills;[3] these disadvantages tended to persist throughout their school career and afterwards, when they started to look for jobs. Similar problems arose with the children of couples who, out of economic necessity, were both working. The present generation of Afro-Caribbean children entering primary school, however, have no language problems if they have attended a nursery school and are also more likely to have a stable home and to be looked after by their parents in the preschool years; their progress in primary school is now indistinguishable from that of other groups.

Religion

Christianity plays an important part in the life of the Afro-Caribbean community in the United Kingdom. The Afro-Caribbeans have tended to set up their own congregations and have their own clergy. In London and the other larger cities formal Christianity and churchgoing seem to be less popular among adolescents and young adults.

The Rastafarian movement, called after Ras Tafari, who in 1930 became Haile Selassie, emperor of Ethiopia, and died in 1975, has attracted many followers among young Afro-Caribbeans.[4] They believe that Ras Tafari, who claimed descent from Solomon, was the Messiah who will lead them back to Ethiopia, the promised land. The men may wear their hair in long ringlets ("dreadlocks") and wear the "tam," a knitted woollen hat in the Ethiopian colours: red, yellow, and green. The women do not cut their hair, which is worn under a scarf. Marijuana ("ganja") is sometimes used as a means of enlightenment and a health giving drug; there is no evidence that the health of their children is in any way affected. Most Rastafarians are strict vegetarians (vegans); when the diet is strictly observed the children may develop nutritional deficiencies.

Language

In the early days of immigration children who spoke at home what is termed Creole by linguists and patois or dialect by Afro-Caribbeans[2] had considerable difficulties on entry to school, but this is no longer so as the present generation of preschool children is usually fluent in the local form of English.

Medical conditions found in the children

Sickle cell disease

In sickle cell disease the red blood cells contain an abnormal haemoglobin (HbS), which causes them to form a sickle shape when exposed to low oxygen tension (fig. 1). Sickle cells aggregate

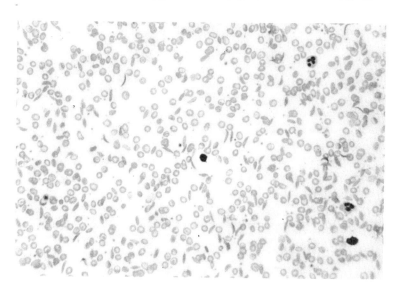

FIG 1—*Blood film of patient with sickle cell disease (by courtesy of Dr J C Sharp).*

in the microcirculation, causing infarction, and have an increased fragility and shortened life, resulting in chronic haemolytic anaemia. The heterozygous sickle cell trait (HbAS), in which there are no symptoms under normal conditions, should be distinguished from the homozygous sickle cell anaemia (HbSS), which is usually severe, occasionally disabling, and sometimes fatal, though a few patients inexplicably have few symptoms (table I shows the distinction between sickle cell trait and sickle cell anaemia). Sickle cell C (HbSC) disease is less common than homozygous sickle cell anaemia and is in general less severe. Homozygous HbCC disease is very rare and presents no special problems, apart from mild anaemia, since there is neither sickling nor haemolysis.

Figure 2 shows the geographical distribution of the sickle cell gene.

Outside Africa the distribution corresponds to that of people of African origin who were dispersed by the slave trade to the West Indies and America; secondary migration has occurred recently to the United Kingdom[1] (fig 3) and elsewhere. The sickle cell gene also occurs in the indigenous population of the north coast of the Mediterranean, Saudi Arabia, round the Persian Gulf, and in some parts of India, mainly in aboriginal tribes; the Arab-Indian form of sickle cell anaemia is less severe than in the African form.

Antenatal screening of all pregnant women, and if necessary of their husbands, should be done in areas with a high proportion of Afro-Caribbeans or a mixed population. Where there is a possibiliy of a homozygous fetus first trimester chorionic villus biopsy should be offered, though the extreme variability in severity of the homozygous state makes advice on testing and termination difficult. Couples who already have a severely affected child are more likely to accept prenatal testing and termination, as subsequent homozygous children are also likely to be severely affected. Cord

TABLE I—*Distinction between sickle cell trait and sickle cell anaemia*

	Symptoms	Anaemia	Jaundice	Splenomegaly	Peripheral film	Sickle cell test
Sickle cell trait	None	None	None	None	Normal	Positive
Sickle cell anaemia	Usually severe	Severe Hb 7-10 g/dl in a stable state	Usually	Yes (up to 8-10 years)	Sickle cells and target cells	Positive

59

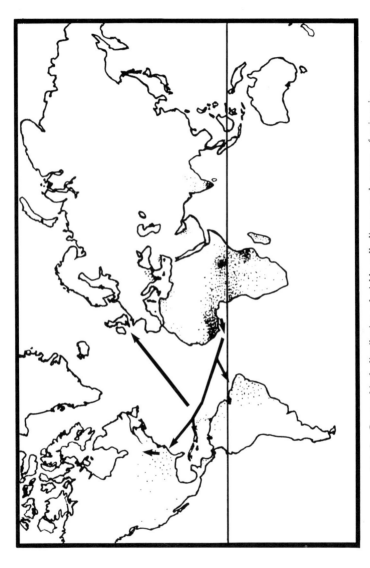

FIG 2—*Geographical distribution of sickle cell disease and routes of migration. Reproduced with permission of author and publisher from Serjeant GR, Sickle Cell Disease. Oxford: Oxford Medical Publications, 1988.*

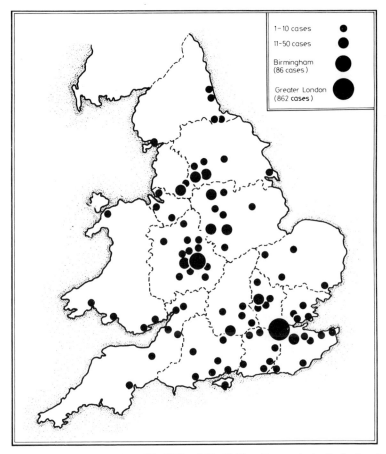

FIG 3—*Davis L R, Huekins E R, White S M. Sickle cell anaemia in England and Wales.* Br Med J *1981; 283: 1519–21. (Reproduced with permission of the authors.)*

blood from *all* infants in a high risk community (see above) should also be tested; the elution of blood spots from cord blood, from a "Guthrie" card is now being tried out in some centres. The children who are heterozygous (sickle cell trait, HbAS) will not develop symptoms, but their parents should be told of the diagnosis and its benign outlook. Infants who are homozygous (HbSS) usually develop symptoms of sickle cell anaemia after the age of 3–4 months and should be carefully followed up from birth at a special clinic, and their parents should be fully informed about

61

the care of their child. The sickle cell test does not yield positive results until the age of 3–4 months, and a positive test does not distinguish between sickle cell trait and sickle cell anaemia (table I); all patients, therefore, showing positive results should be investigated initially by a competent haematologist.

In infancy—The infant presents at the age of 3–4 months with failure to thrive, recurrent infections, anaemia, jaundice, and splenomegaly (the spleen usually shrinks progressively and becomes impalpable by the age of 8–10 years).

Acute illness at any age over 4 months—Whatever the diagnosis a child who is acutely ill and is known to have, or is suspected of having, sickle cell anaemia should be admitted to hospital immediately. Acute pneumococcal infections, pneumonia, septicaemia, and meningitis are particularly common. Severe sickling crises may be precipitated by any acute infection, acidosis, dehydration, hypoxia, trauma, exposure to cold, or by a general anaesthetic if special precautions are not taken. Severe shock may develop, particularly in young children with enlarged spleens when sequestration of blood occurs in the spleen. Aplastic crises are not common and may be due to infections with parvovirus,[5] sometimes affecting several members of the same family simultaneously; megaloblastic crises due to dietary folic acid deficiency, however, are common in the West Indies and may occur in Britain in children on inadequate diets (see page 57 under Religion). The "bilateral chest syndrome" and extensive mesenteric infarction may occasionally prove fatal.

Jaundice may be due to: haemolysis in a sickling crisis; to hepatitis A or B, which may also provoke sickling; hepatic crises with pooling and sickling in the liver and signs of obstructive jaundice; or, in children over 10 years, to obstruction by bile pigment gall stones.

Localised infarction producing pain and swelling—In infants the fingers and toes are often affected ("dactylitis," and "hand-foot" syndrome). Disease of the mesenteric vessels may mimic an abdominal emergency. Hemiplegia or other neurological infarction syndromes are particularly disabling. Haematuria occurs but is rare, as is priapism.

Sickle cell disease and the family doctor.

The family doctor should ensure that all his Afro-Caribbean and African patients are tested for sickle cell disease, and those with a positive result and members of their families should be further investigated. About one in 10 Afro-Caribbeans have the sickle cell trait and about one in 400 infants will have sickle cell anaemia. Anyone with sickle cell anaemia should wear a Medialert necklace or bracelet, and the parents of an affected child should contact a local branch of the Organisation of Sickle Cell Anaemia Research or the Sickle Cell Society (see Useful addresses).

Prophylactic dental care is important and should be encouraged. When this is local policy parents should be strongly advised to have their children immunised against pneumococcal infection (Pneumovax, Morson) with two injections, at 6 and 18 months and to maintain their daily prophylactic penicillin. Folic acid supplements should be maintained if this is local policy, though present evidence suggests that in Britain aplastic crises are more likely to be due to infections with parvovirus,[5] while megaloblastic crises due to folic acid deficiency are rare. Oral iron should not be prescribed for anaemic patients in whom iron deficiency has not been proved. Analgesia at home, for painful crises, should be confined to paracetamol and strictly limited supplies of dihydrocodeine (DF118), as this is potentially habit forming. Dipipanone, dextropropoxyphene with paracetamol (Distalgesic), and similar habit forming drugs should be prescribed only in hospital or in exceptional circumstances at home. Flying in commercial aircraft, which are normally pressurised at 2300 m (7000 ft), constitutes a risk to those with sickle cell anaemia but not to those with the trait. The airline should be informed well before the flight and the availability of an oxygen supply other than the emergency one should be discussed; splenic infarction appears to be the commonest complication of flying, and those who have previously experienced an infarct are likely to do so again.

Haemoglobin SC disease and sickle cell thalassaemia

Haemoglobin SC disease and sickle cell thalassaemia are much less common than sickle cell anaemia,[6] while HbCC disease is extremely rare. Haemoglobin SC disease and sickle cell thalassaemia have less severe symptoms than does homozygous sickle cell disease. HbCC disease presents as mild anaemia.

Glucose 6 phosphate dehydrogenase (G6PD) deficiency

Glucose 6 phosphate dehydrogenase deficiency, inherited through an X-linked intermediate gene and therefore seen predominantly in men, occurs in the fairly benign African form in Afro-Caribbeans. Homozygous women are not uncommon and may be as severely affected as are the men; rarely, a heterozygous woman may be mildly affected clinically. Favism, an acute and severe haemolysis due to contact with the broad bean (*Vicia faba*) or its pollen, appears to be confined to Mediterranean and Far Eastern types (for further discussion see chapter 5: Families from the Mediterranean and Aegean and chapter 6: Chinese and Vietnamese families). In affected subjects the red blood cells haemolyse after the patient has taken certain drugs (table II) or under conditions of severe hypoxia or acidosis, particularly in diabetic ketoacidosis and during acute infections such as hepatitis. Clinically, G6PD defficiency takes two forms: jaundice in the neonatal period or an acute self limiting haemolysis precipitated by one of

TABLE II—*Drugs likely to cause haemolysis in G6PD deficiency**

Antimalarials	Primaquine
	Pamaquine
	Pentaquine
Sulphonamides	Sulphanilamide
	Sulphacetamide
	Sulphapyridine
	Sulphamethoxazole (in Bactrim and Septrin)
	Silver sulphadiazine
	(surface application for burns)
Sulphones	Dapsone (in Maloprim, prophylaxis for malaria)
	Thiazolesulphone
Nitrofurans	Nitrofurantoin (Furadantin)
Analgesics	Acetanilide
Miscellaneous	Methylene blue
	Nalidixic acid (Negram)
	Naphthalene
	Niridazole
	Phenylhydrazine
	Toluidine blue
	Trinitrotoluene

Table modified from: Wintrobe M M, Lee G R, Boggs D R, *et al. Clinical Hematology.* 8th ed. Philadelphia: Lea and Febiger, 1981:792, with permission from authors and publishers.
*Different authors give slightly different lists.

the drugs listed in table II. In the African form spontaneous jaundice without drug contact may develop in the full term infant as well as in the preterm infant, usually on the second or third day of life, reaching a maximum on or around the third to the sixth day and subsiding by the end of the first week. Infants may also become jaundiced after contact with one of the offending drugs through the placenta, in breast milk, as part of treament, after applications to the cord (usually menthol preparations), or after contact with babies' clothes impregnated with naphthalene (mothballs). The timing of jaundice obviously depends on the time of contact. In Britain jaundice from G6PD deficiency is not common in Afro-Caribbean infants, but the diagnosis must nevertheless be considered when there is no obvious cause for non-obstructive jaundice. Other factors such as incompatibility of blood groups, sepsis, or reabsorption of extravasated blood may be contributory factors.

In the older child or adult a sudden haemolysis lasting about 36 hours may develop after drug contact but is less severe, because haemolysis is self limiting, than in the Mediterranean and Far Eastern forms; jaundice is not evident at the time of the haemolysis because the process is so quick. Deaths from haemolysis are rare in Afro-Caribbeans (for further discussion and a table showing the differences between the three types of G6PD deficiency see chapters 5: Families from the Mediterranean and Aegean and 6: Chinese and Vietnamese families).

Lactase deficiency

Lactase deficiency (lactose malabsorption, intolerance, maldigestion) has not been studied in the Afro-Caribbean population in Britain, but is present in about 70% of black Americans over the age of 6–7 years.[8] For fuller discussion see chapter 6: Chinese and Vietnamese families.

Acquired diseases

In the neonatal period subaponeurotic haemorrhage appears to be more common in infants of Afro-Caribbean or African origin; though the reason for this is not known. Neonatal jaundice may occur (for further discussion see G6PD deficiency), and the breast enlargement that is sometimes seen in the first week of life may persist in some Afro-Caribbean girls until the age of 4–5 years (see also below, under Premature thelarche).

During infancy and childhood the following conditions may occur.

Umbilical hernia is common in Afro-Caribbean and African children; if large or persistent (until the age of 3–4 years) it may require operation.

Keloid formation is more likely to develop in postoperative or post-traumatic scars or after burns than in other racial groups.

Nutritional deficiencies—Normally Afro-Caribbean and African children are well nourished, though a mild iron deficiency anaemia is common. Children brought up in a Rastafarian family on a strict vegetarian diet may develop nutritional rickets,[9] and there is a risk of megaloblastic anaemia and glossitis due to deficiency of vitamin B_{12} or folic acid.[10 11]

Premature thelarche (premature development of breasts) seems to occur more often in Afro-Caribbean girls than in other ethnic groups. The enlargement may occur as early as 4–5 years but is not accompanied by other evidence of puberty or signs of endocrine disease. Provided that the breast enlargement remains an isolated symptom there is no reason for anxiety or specialised investigation. Such children should, however, be seen at least once by a paediatric endocrinologist and should then be examined regularly until normal puberty is established. No treatment is available or is required except reassurance.

Premature pubarche (premature development of pubic hair) also appears to be fairly common in Afro-Caribbean girls. As with premature thelarche there is no cause for anxiety or for endocrine investigation if there is no evidence of endocrine disease or other signs of incipient puberty. The management is as for premature development of the breasts.

Emoional, social, and school problems

Baby minding and deprivation—The slow development of a deprived child may be due solely to the unstimulating environment provided by a baby minder; the circumstances that lead to this situation have been described previously.

Poor school progress may be due initially to deprivation but is now more likely to be related to poor self esteem and a sense of hopelessness induced by the probability of unemployment on leaving school.

Parental attitudes to punishment—Physical punishment as a form of parental discipline has traditionally been used by Afro-Caribbean families. The use of a belt or strap, usually by the father, does not indicate a disturbed family relationship or a sadistic parental attitude and should not normally be dealt with as "child abuse" unless there is severe or repeated injury.

African families

Most African families in Britain are West Africans from Nigeria or Ghana. They usually come to Britain for further education or to obtain a professional qualification. If both parents are studying, as is often the case, the need to complete their course successfully is in competition with traditional expectations, their own and those of their families at home, that they should have a child. This may result in their child being sent, often when very young, to a baby minder during the day; or fostering may be arranged on a long term basis, often with a white couple. The problems of a Nigerian couple in London have been described by Buchi Emecheta in *Second Class Citizen.*[12]

Religion—In Ghana about 60% of the population are Christians of various denominations; the remainder are Moslems. Dietary restrictions on pork and pork products are similar to those for Asian Moslems. In Nigeria also Islam and Christianity are the most important religions.

Language—The main languages in Nigeria are Yoruba, Ibo, and Hausa; in Ghana Akan, Gā, and Ewe. In both countries English is the second language. Language is unlikely to be a problem to a child who has been with an English speaking baby minder or whose parents have found them a place at a day nursery. In areas where there are many children for whom English is the second language special attention is given at entry to school; but language difficulties are, nevertheless, not uncommon, particularly in Nigerian children. Difficulties may arise for a child who has remained in Africa with grandparents and come to Britain at the age of 8–9

67

years, to a new country and to parents and perhaps siblings who are complete strangers.

Medical conditions found in the children

Genetically determined conditions

Sickle cell disease, HbSC disease, HbS thalassaemia, HbCC disease, and G6PD deficiency all occur in African children with the same symptoms as those described for Afro-Caribbeans. In west Africans the incidence of sickle cell trait is, however, about one in five of the population, and therefore one in 100–200 infants can be expected to develop symptoms of sickle cell anaemia. HbSC is commoner in west Africans than in Afro-Caribbeans. Lactase deficiency is present in over 70% of adults and older children (the exact age at which lactase activity declines in these groups is not clear) in the parts of Africa from which most Africans in Britain originate.[8]

Acquired diseases

For subaponeurotic haemorrhage, neonatal jaundice, umbilical hernia, and keloid formation see under the paragraphs dealing with Afro-Caribbean children.

Schistosomiasis—Both *Schistosoma haematobium* and *S mansoni* are common throughout rural Africa and are acquired by contact with infected water from rivers but rarely infect children before they can walk independently. *S haematobium* infection should be suspected in children who have recently been in Africa if they develop recurrent attacks of haematuria, with dysuria and frequency, or an apparently straightforward attack of acute pyelonephritis that fails to improve. Infection with *S mansoni* is more likely to produce chronic diarrhoea with blood and mucus in the stool. Both types of infection can produce malaise without localised symptoms, with or without hepatosplenomegaly. A child in whom schistosomiasis is suspected should be referred to someone with experience of this condition.

Malaria is common in most parts of Africa, and chloroquine resistance is particularly common in Tanzania and the coastal regions of Kenya. Children should be tested for G6PD deficiency before being given primaquine (for further discussion of malaria and map see chapter 4: Asian families II: conditions that may be found in the children.

Hookworm (ankylostomiasis) should be considered in a child who has recently arrived from Africa and has an unexplained or iron resistant anaemia. Ankylostomiasis is unlikely in infants, town dwellers, or children from hot, dry parts of Africa (for further discussion of hookworm see chapter 4: Asian families II: conditions that may be found in the children.

Female circumcision and infibulation—In Britain only late complications of the most extensive form of female circumcision, the pharaonic type (infibulation), are likely to be seen. Though widely practised in Africa, it is not performed in Ghana but is common in Nigeria, in both Moslem and Christian families. Regrettably, female circumcision has also been performed in private clinics in London. The operation, which is often carried out before the age of 10 days or as late as 7–8 years consists of removing the clitoris and labia minora and all or part of the labia majora; the cut edges are held together but a small aperture is left for the passage of urine and menstrual discharge. In Nigeria a modified operation is sometimes performed with removal of the clitoris and trimming of the labia minora round the clitoris. The late complications that may arise are: urinary tract infection, a poor urinary stream related to obstruction from meatal scarring or urethral stricture, complete or almost complete labial fusion, rectovaginal fistulae, implantation dermoids, keloid scarring, and in older girls, introital stenosis.

1 Davis L R, Heukins E R, White S M. Survey of sickle cell disease in England and Wales. *Br Med J* 1981; **283**:1519–21.
2 Edwards V K. *The West Indian language issue in British schools*. London: Routledge and Kegan Paul, 1979.
3 Scarrs S, Caparalo B K, Ferdman B M, Tower R B, Caplan J. Developmental status and school achievements of minority and non-minority children from birth to 18 years in a British midlands town. *British Journal of Developmental Psychology* 1983; **1**:31–48.
4 Springer L, Thomas J. Rastafarians in Britain: a preliminary study of their food habits and beliefs. *Hum Nutr Appl Nutr* 1983; **37**:120–7.
5 Serjeant G R, Topley J M, Mason K, *et al*. Outbreak of aplastic crises in sickle cell anaemia associated with a parvovirus-like agent. *Lancet* 1981; **ii**:595–7.
6 Mann J R. Sickle cell haemoglobinopathies in England. *Arch Dis Child* 1981; **56**:676–83.
7 Gibbs W H, Gray R, Lowry M. Glucose-6-phosphate dehydrogenase deficiency and neonatal jaundice in Jamaica. *Br J Haematol* 1979; **43**:263–74.

8 Scrimshaw N, Murray E B. The acceptability of milk and milk products in populations with a high prevalence of lactose intolerance. *Am J Clin Nutr* 1988. **48** suppl:1083–159.

9 Ward P S, Drakeford J P, Milton J, James J A. Nutritional rickets in Rastafarian children. *Br Med J* 1982; **285**:1242–3.

10 Campbell M, Lofters W S, Gibbs W N. Rastafarianism and the vegans syndrome. *Br Med J* 1982; **285**:1617–8.

11 Close G C. Rastafarianism and the vegans syndrome. *Br Med J* 1982; **286**:473.

12 Emecheta B. *Second Class Citizen*. Glasgow: Fontana and Collins, 1974.

Further reading

Ellis J. *West African Families in Britain*. London: Routledge and Kegan Paul, 1978.

Fleming A F, ed. *Sickle cell disease*. Edinburgh: Churchill Livingstone, 1982.

Anionwu E, Hall J. *Handbook on sickle cell disease: a guide for families*. London: Sickle Cell Society, 1983.

Lehmann H, Huntsman R G. *Man's haemoglobins*. Amsterdam and Oxford: North Holland Publishing Company, 1974.

Pollak M. The care of immigrant children. In: Hart C, ed. *Child care in general practice*. 2nd ed. Edinburgh: Churchill Livingstone, 1982.

Useful addresses for advice and counselling

London

Sickle Cell Society, Green Lodge, Barrett's Green Road, London NW10 (01 961 7795/8346)

Lambeth Sickle Cell Centre, 2 Stockwell Road, London SW9 9EN (01 737 3588)

Sickle Cell Centre, Royal Northern Hospital, Holloway Road, London N7 (01 272 7777, ext 351)

City and Hackney Sickle Cell Centre, St Leonard's Hospital, Nuttall Street, London N1 5LZ (01 739 8484)

George Marsh Sickle Cell and Thalassaemia Centre, St Ann's Hospital, St Ann's Road, London N15 3TH (01 800 0121, ext 4230 or 809 1797)

St Thomas's Hospital Community Midwives Office, London SE1 7EH (01 928 9292, ext 2257/3123)

Organisation for Sickle Cell Anaemia Research, 22 Pellatt Grove, London N22 5PL (01 889 4844/3300)

Birmingham

Carnegie Centre for Community Service, Hunter's Road, Hockley, Birmingham (021 554 3899, ext 236)

Cardiff

Butetown Health Centre, Lourdon Square Docks, Cardiff (0222 488027)

Liverpool

Liverpool Sickle Cell Centre, Abercromby Health Centre, Grove Street, Liverpool 8 (051 708 9370)

Manchester

Moss Side Health Centre, Monton Street, Manchester 14 (061 226 8972/5031)

Index